*Improving American Indian
Health Care*

Improving American Indian Health Care

THE WESTERN CHEROKEE EXPERIENCE

C. WILLIAM STEELER

EDITED BY
GARY W. SHANNON
AND
RASHID L. BASHSHUR

UNIVERSITY OF OKLAHOMA PRESS : NORMAN

Publication of this book is made possible through the generosity of Edith Gaylord Harper.

Library of Congress Cataloging-in-Publication Data

Steeler, C. William, 1948–1992.
    Improving American Indian health care : the western Cherokee experience / C. William Steeler ; edited by Gary W. Shannon and Rashid L. Bashshur.
        p. cm.
    Includes bibliographical references and index.
    ISBN 0-8061-3356-2 (alk. paper)
    1. Indians of North America—Health and hygiene.   2. Cherokee Indians—Medical care.   I. Shannon, Gary William.   II. Bashshur, Rashid, 1933–   III. Title.

RA448.5.I5 S74 2001
362.1'089'9755—dc21

                                                    2001027568

Contents

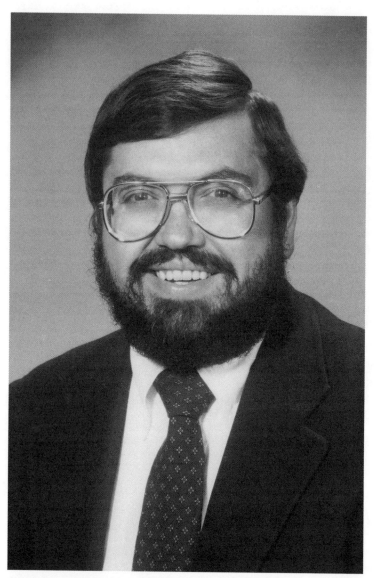

C. William Steeler. Photo by Studio Fauré, Chantilly.

In Memory of C. William Steeler (1948–1992)

Bill Steeler died without warning in his sleep on April 30, 1992, at his home in Gouvieux, France. Born in Tulsa, Oklahoma, he received a B.B.A. in 1973 and an M.H.S.A. in 1976 from Oklahoma State University. He served first as an economist and later as an executive officer with the Indian Health Service from 1978 to 1984. Bill became Director of Operations for the U.S. Indian Health Service in Portland, Oregon, prior to becoming Executive Director for Health of the Cherokee Nation of Oklahoma. At the time of his death, he was Director of Primary Health Care Programs for His Highness the Aga Khan's Health Services, in Aiglemont, France, a position he had held since 1986. In 1990 Bill received his Dr.P.H. from the University of Michigan School of Public Health. His dissertation was entitled *Selected Health Policy Issues Among Native Americans.*

Bill was known as a widely read, thoughtful man; his dedication to the development of people and the improvement of lives reflected both his humanity and his understanding of the importance of human resources to the success of health programs. He felt a kinship between the values of the Cherokee culture from which he had come and those of the Ismaili communities that he came to serve. Bill possessed both a deep understanding of the spiritual purpose of his work and the dedication and competence necessary to do it well. His work among both communities in the design of health systems pointed the way toward the rational linkage of primary health care and curative services with community development.

Bill was recognized for his sustained efforts to improve health conditions through grass roots community involvement, for his unselfish commitment, and for his dedication and hard work. Classmates at the University of Michigan remember him as a natural leader who was respected and admired. His friends and colleagues remember him fondly for his many fine qualities—his ever present smile, his keen sense of humor, and his strong sense of purpose.

Bill's sudden, unexpected, and premature death ended a life dedicated to human service and an exceptional career dedicated to developing and directing health care improvement among deserving communities. It also took from us too soon a valued friend and family member. It did not and cannot take, however, his memory—to which this volume is dedicated.

Preface

This book is dedicated to the memory of C. William Steeler. It derives from his doctoral dissertation, completed at the University of Michigan School of Public Health. We have added an introductory chapter, which provides an overview of Cherokee history, and a brief epilogue. In addition, we have updated some sections with more recent literature, statistics, and legislation pertaining to the Indian health experience generally and the Cherokee experience specifically. The vast majority and essence of the work, however, is that of Bill Steeler.

The book addresses some basic health policy concerns of Native Americans by describing the response of the Cherokee Nation of Oklahoma (Nation) to a series of three policy issues directly concerned with health and health care. The first issue involves a change in health care eligibility regulations proposed by the Indian Health Service. Next addressed is the importance to Native American communities of developing a more direct and communal sense of responsibility for the health status of individuals within the community as well as for the health of the community in general, within the context of a shared responsibility with the federal government. The third concern is the perceived need for communities to develop and facilitate coordination among providers of health services, inasmuch as such coordination affects both health status and social and economic development.

Each of the three issues is outlined, and subsequently the process of response development and the actual response to each issue by the Nation are described. The solutions and approaches here are not meant to be singularly prescriptive or limited to one setting. Rather, we hope, as did Bill Steeler, that the narratives will inform and generate debate within the leadership and membership of all Native American tribal

organizations toward the development of long-term policies and strategies aimed at achieving the highest possible level of health for Native
Americans. The case studies of the Cherokee Nation's experience may
provide useful models for other tribal organizations facing similar problems related to poor health conditions and limited resources. The challenge lies in finding ways to utilize available external and internal
resources, including self-reliance, mobilization of community resources,
and a sense of personal and community responsibility for individuals'
health and well-being, in order to maximize long-term health benefits.

Tribal organizations concerned with health care issues may benefit
by sharing experiences in a constructive and supportive way. When
given the opportunity to see how others have addressed health policy
issues, tribal governments may choose to adopt or adapt those approaches
particularly suitable to their own circumstances, while retaining control
over their internal affairs. When lessons are learned from actual experiences of other Native American groups, they may be all the more com-
pelling. This work is intended to enlighten Native Americans and the
general population to the problems facing Native Americans in the pursuit of improved health status.

Bill Steeler was particularly well-placed and well-informed with regard
to the issues discussed in this book. He served as Executive Director for
Health of the Cherokee Nation of Oklahoma. He also served as an executive staff member of the Indian Health Service during the development of the specific situations that form the basis of this volume. He
participated in the enactment of the policies and responses described
herein. Because of Bill's proximity to the people and the issues addressed,
his interpretations of the Nation's ultimate responses and his conclusions necessarily must be subjected to close scrutiny. On the other hand,
few could have been better situated to gain insight into these issues. The
success of this work rests upon the interest it generates in policy discussion among members of Native American organizations, the body
politic, and the general population.

The underlying theme of this work is the proactive and self-reliant
approach adopted by the government of the Cherokee Nation to improve
the health status of its people. This movement began shortly after enactment of the Indian Self-Determination and Education Assistance Act of
1975 (P.L. 93-638), which affirmed the rights of Indian tribes to manage

their internal affairs. Specifically, the Act gave tribes the option of staffing and managing health programs in their communities and provided the funding for improvement of tribal capability to contract under the Act. The 1976 Indian Health Care Improvement Act, P.L. 94-437, was intended to raise the health status of Native Americans to a level equal to that of the general population.

The concepts of activism and self-reliance in health care affairs refer here to the Nation's assumption of responsibility for improving the health of its citizens through its own communal organizations and leadership. The Cherokee Nation initiated programs for long-term development and health improvement based on this concept of self-reliance.

Improving American Indian Health Care

Introduction

The central concerns of this book are the health and health care of the Native American population. More precisely, the book focuses on deficiencies in the health of Native Americans as compared to the general population and on attempts to resolve problems related to health status through improvement of health services delivery. Several indicators point to continuing lower health status among Native Americans. For instance, for the reporting period 1986–88, the age-adjusted mortality rate (all causes) for Native Americans in the Indian Health Service (IHS) area, which is comprised of twelve area offices whose health care responsibilities extend to all or parts of thirty-four states (known as the Reservation States), was 665.8 (rate per 100,000) compared to 535.5 for the general U.S. population. Figures for 1989–91 indicate the age-adjusted mortality rate (all causes) for Native Americans residing in the IHS service area was 585.2 (rate per 100,000 population) compared to 520.2 for the general population. However, when the mortality rate is adjusted to account for the underreporting of Indian race on death certificates, the rate becomes 713.9. This is a mortality rate 37 percent greater than the rate for the general population.

There remain significant differences between the age-adjusted mortality rate of Native Americans living in the Reservation States and that of the general population, for a number of causes. In 1990, for example, for Indians the mortality rate from alcoholism was 630 percent greater than that of the general population; tuberculosis, 580 percent greater; chronic liver disease and cirrhosis, 352 percent greater; diabetes mellitus, 232 percent greater; accidents, 232 percent greater; suicide and homicide, about 80 percent greater (IHS 1994, table 4.9). So the differentials in mortality rates for tuberculosis, alcoholism, and diabetes mellitus between Native Americans and the general population actually increased between 1987 and 1990 (U.S. Congress 1992). However, in 1990 the death rate from malignant neoplasms was 18 percent lower for Native Americans than for the general population (Indian Health Service 1994). The death rates for major cardiovascular diseases and chronic obstructive pulmonary diseases were slightly lower than those of the general population as well.

Meanwhile, life expectancy of Native Americans continues to increase at a rate faster than that of the general population. In 1980, life expectancy at birth for Native Americans was 71.1 years (67.1 years for males and 75.1 years for females), an increase of 19 percent since 1950. Despite these gains, life expectancy continued to lag behind that of the white population (74.4 years for both sexes, 70.7 years for males, and 78.1 years for females) (IHCIA 1992, 94).

Thus, it would appear that some improvements in the health status of Native Americans have been accomplished. But it is obvious that the most recent effort to improve the health status of Native Americans, begun with the enactment of the Indian Health Care Improvement Act in 1976, is not complete. In 1992 the Select Senate Committee on Indian Affairs revised and reauthorized extension of the Improvement Act through fiscal year 2000. This would enable the IHS and the tribal governments to achieve the goals and objectives stipulated for Native Americans in *Healthy People 2000: National Health Promotion and Disease Prevention Objectives* (DHHS Publication No. 91-50212). Developed by the Department of Health and Human Services, this document set forth thirty-one health status objectives targeted specifically at Native Americans. The overall goal was to upgrade the health status of Native Americans to the level of the general population.

There is a need to analyze the basic policies and programs that have been put in place for the purpose of improving the health status of Native Americans and to determine the most effective means through which improvements in their health status are to be achieved. Policies that govern the programs are formulated at four levels of government: federal, state, local, and tribal. However, there is generally little coordination or integration among these levels of government. Moreover, the responsibility for providing the services necessary to improve health conditions rests with an assortment of programs. At the federal level, the Indian Health Service of the Department of Health and Human Services, established in 1955, holds the primary responsibility. Another major department at the federal level is the Bureau of Indian Affairs (BIA) of the Department of the Interior. The variety of agencies at the state and local levels increases, and the organizational structure of units concerned with Native American affairs varies from state to state. In some states there is an Office of Indian Affairs housed within one of the human service departments.

The mutual interdependence model has been advanced to help resolve conflicting understandings and expectations about the cooperative process by articulating a new, overarching view of them relative to processes and roles of two interacting parties. The mutual interdependence model fosters cooperation by building common understandings and expectations between public policymakers, legislators, and the target community (Bennett 1993). The obstacles and issues facing Native Americans in their pursuit of independence, within the context of mutual interdependence, are numerous and complex. This book identifies several problems and illustrates the approaches taken to ameliorate them by the Cherokee Nation of Oklahoma in hopes that the Cherokee experience may prove applicable and useful in other Native American communities. We join others who postulate that an examination of the Cherokee experience provides a foundation for understanding the relationships between the United States and the indigenous first nations of North America. Further, the principles and persistent efforts of the Cherokee can serve as a prototype for other Indian (and non-Indian) groups in the quest to maintain and expand fundamental human rights (Norgen 1996).

CHAPTER ONE

The Cherokee Nation

Whereas, it being the anxious desire of the Government of the United States to secure the Cherokee nation of Indians . . . a permanent home, and which shall, under the most solemn guarantees of the United States, be and remain theirs forever—a home that shall never, in all future time, be embarrassed by having extended around it lines, or placed over it the jurisdiction of any of the limits of any existing Territory or States . . . the parties hereto do hereby conclude the following Articles.

TREATY OF 1828

There are approximately 1.5 million Native Americans and Alaska Natives in all Indian Health Service Areas. Of these, about one third live on reservations or historic trust lands, and about one half live in urban areas (IHS 1994, Table 2.1). The Oklahoma Indian Health Service Area includes about 300,000 people. This is the largest number of Native Americans concentrated in any single Area. The limestone face of Oklahoma's Ozark Plateau, a place of spring-fed creeks and riffled rivers, is Indian country, but it is not a reservation. This is the home of the Cherokee Nation, a federally recognized sovereign nation established and maintained by treaty with the United States through much of the nineteenth century. At that time, before the treaties were broken and the territory opened to statehood, Oklahoma was the refuge for vestiges of more than sixty displaced tribes. The Cherokees were the most numerous, and their predominance among Native Americans continues in the region to this day (Norman 1995). Now, in fourteen counties of northeastern Oklahoma, about 165,000 full and mixed-blood Cherokee count themselves members of the Cherokee Nation, which has been uniquely successful among Native American tribes in the administration of its own affairs.

A BRIEF HISTORY OF THE CHEROKEE

The ancient history of the Cherokee remains cloaked in mystery, debate and speculation. On the other hand, the past two hundred years of their odyssey has been well documented. The more recent history of the Cherokee is treated in detail elsewhere (see, for example, King 1979 and McLoughlin 1993), but a brief synopsis of the recent history is given here in order to provide a contextual framework for the discussion of health policy issues confronting the Cherokee Nation and to give insight into the response of the Nation to these issues. This synopsis also provides insight into the historical response of the Cherokee to threats to their society.

Though the prehistory of the Cherokee remains a matter of debate, linguistic evidence suggests they shared an early association with the Iroquois nations of the Tuscarora, Seneca, Cayuga, and Oneida. However, linguistic comparisons show that Cherokee is quite distinct from the other Iroquois languages, indicating if not an earlier, certainly a more complete separation (Lounsbury 1961; Coe 1961). One writer has suggested that the early Iroquois nations were comprised of a "lone southern (Cherokee) branch and a large northern trunk" (Lounsbury 1961).

The linguistic differences as well as the diversity of the traditional Cherokee practices and customs have led to considerable speculation as to when and where the tribes originally separated. There is some evidence of a southward migration from the eastern seaboard (Woodward 1963, 19). Delaware tradition mentions a prehistoric migration of the Cherokees with whom they fought for many years. Some speculate that the prehistoric Cherokee occupied a portion of the Great Lakes region, and still others suggest the Cherokee originated in the Orinoco and Amazon river basins of South America. Whether they migrated from the north, west, east, or even south, it is generally agreed that the arrival of the Cherokee into the Southern Appalachian region occurred only shortly before European contact. Apparently this coincided with the arrival of De Soto in their country in 1540.

Territory occupied by the Cherokee at the beginning of the eighteenth century may be divided into four major areas. The lower settlement of Cherokee occupied relatively flat lands on the banks of the Tugaloo and Keeowee Rivers, in what is today northwestern South Carolina. The middle settlement was situated among the mountains of western North Carolina. The remaining Overhill and Valley settlements were located in eastern Tennessee and the extreme western tip of North Carolina, respectively (Fogelson and Kutsche 1961). These areas comprised the core of Cherokee settlement. However, the Cherokee dominated an even larger area extending into regions of present day Virginia, West Virginia, Kentucky, Alabama, and Georgia.

Once known to others as the "warlords of the southern mountains," the Cherokees called themselves the *Ani Yun wiay*, meaning the leading or the Principal People (Norman 1995). In truculent times, they fought with their neighbors, including the Choctaw and Creek. They fought as well against the English, against the New World French and the early European settlers in America. As a relatively unassimilated aboriginal culture about 1700, the Cherokee quickly adopted much from European material culture and gradually adopted social and political ideas as well. They built European-style homes and farmsteads, laid out European-style fields and farms, developed a written language, established a newspaper, and wrote a constitution. The rise of the Cherokee State in the mid-1700s was an instance of independent communities or villages joining voluntarily (Gearing 1961).

Cherokee villagers consciously distinguished between two categories of village tasks; and villagers organized themselves differently when they attended the tasks in each category. The Red Organization executed political control of towns during military emergencies. The tasks of officials in the Red, or War, organization included war and negotiation with foreign powers in matters of trade. These were coordinated by a command structure under the settlement or "town" war chief, the Red War Chief or Raven. Election to this position was based on an individual's notable exploits as a warrior.

Officials in the White Organization had responsibility during peacetime for ceremonials and councils. And they had responsibility for directing communal farming (Thomas 1961). The responsibilities were coordinated by a voluntary consensus created through the influence of the elders in their respective clans. In turn, the elders were under the leadership of the town's priest (White) chief, who was both the symbol of town harmony and the major overseer of that harmony (Gearing 1961). It is reported that communal decisions were generally unanimous and that direct coercion or "overactive" leadership was strongly devalued (Fogelson and Kutsche 1961). Throughout the history of the Cherokee, there has been a decided disinclination toward the elevation of the individual (Fogelson 1961).

Thus, the physical and spiritual center of eighteenth century Cherokee life was the town (Goggin 1961). The typical town of this period was a small settlement consisting of between 200 and 325 people. More important towns and the "sacred mother towns" were much larger with perhaps 600 people, while the smallest towns had populations of less than 100.

The lack of a strong centralized organization and authority among the Cherokee towns was apparently frustrating to early Colonial administrators desiring to develop "nationwide" treaties (Fogelson and Kutsche 1961). The rise of the Cherokee State in the mid-1700s was an instance of independent, proximal towns joining voluntarily. An important factor in this cooperative effort was the pressure and duress deriving from the new colony of South Carolina. The colony treated the independent Cherokee towns as a single political unit. Thus, reprisals for events that occurred between members of one town and colonists would be administered to other towns. The Cherokee in one village had no control over the behavior of those in other villages, and yet they were held accountable for it (Gearing 1961). During the last part of the eighteenth century, the Cherokee became embroiled in a period of intensive warfare with early American settlers, and their political unification in response to the advancing white frontier increased. In the process, the local towns were gradually stripped of their autonomy and independence.

After the American Revolution, there was a flood of white migration toward the Cherokee borders. This was a period of almost constant bloodshed and destruction of their towns. The Cherokee sued for peace in 1782 and, subsequently, increased trade and contact accelerated the pace of acculturation with the settlers. By about 1815, Cherokees owned farmsteads in north Georgia and other fertile areas, which rivaled plantations of the whites in sophistication and number of slaves. Many of the Cherokee were educated in American schools and rapidly achieved dominance in the Cherokee political affairs. At the same time, earlier patterns of kinship and religion were crumbling under the weight of missionaries who successfully converted the Cherokee to Christianity. Geographically, the center of educational and missionary activities was concentrated in the southern portions of the Cherokee Nation.

Change in the political structure occurred rapidly. After 1820, the traditional White Organization among the Cherokee was replaced, and the Nation was remodeled into a republic along the lines of the government of the United States. The "invention" of the Sequoyah (George Guess) syllabary/alphabet in 1821 was acclaimed as a tool of progress. Sequoyah, a half-blooded Cherokee, became convinced of the importance of the written language to accumulating and transmitting knowledge. As early as 1809, he began working systematically to develop a written language for the Cherokees, experimenting first with pictographs and then with symbols representing the syllables of the spoken language. Assisted by his daughter, Sequoyah identified the syllables and then adapted letters from English as well as Greek and Hebrew. By 1821, he had perfected 86 letters, representing all the syllables of the Cherokee language. The Cherokee established schools where Sequoyah's alphabet was taught.

The Cherokee could now publish their own books, newspapers, laws, and constitution (Fogelson 1961). Indeed, in 1827 a constitution was ratified which provided for the election of a chief and vice chief. The Nation was divided into election districts. The days of local town autonomy were over, for it was recognized that only a unified national state would be of sufficient strength to battle the U.S. government for retention of ancestral lands within the unmarked borders of the Nation.

National policy to move Indians west of the Mississippi developed after the Louisiana Territory was purchased from the French in 1803. As white settlers moved onto these lands, they pressed the U.S. government to do something to diminish the Indian presence. In 1825 the U.S. government formally adopted a removal policy which was carried out in the 1830s by Presidents Andrew Jackson and Martin Van Buren.

In 1830 Congress passed Andrew Jackson's Indian Removal Act, which directed the executive branch to negotiate for Indian lands. President Jackson was not only a southern slaveholder, but he also fought against the Creek and Seminole Indians in Alabama and Florida, respectively. Freeing the West (then the eastern half of the Mississippi Valley) of Indians so European migrants could settle the land was among his primary goals as president. Indeed, Jackson was instrumental in removing the tribes of the southeastern United States. In part this was done on the grounds that they were "too savage" to live among and compete with whites. According to Jackson, the Indians were "established in the midst of another and a superior race and without appreciating the causes of their inferiority or seeking to control them, they must necessarily yield to the force of circumstances and ere long disappear" (McLoughlin 1993). Indeed, Andrew Jackson's political ascendancy in the 1820s was predicated upon and encouraged a federal policy that replaced an ambivalence toward the Cherokee with a determined program of removal.

The Indian Removal Act, in combination with the discovery of gold and an increasingly untenable position with the state of Georgia, prompted the Cherokee Nation to bring suit in the U.S. Supreme Court. In *Cherokee Nation v. Georgia* (1831), the U.S. Supreme Court, led by Chief Justice John Marshall writing for the majority, held that the Cherokee Nation was "a domestic, dependent nation," and therefore Georgia state law applied to it. While the Cherokees put the emphasis on "nation," the Bureau of Indian Affairs (BIA) put the emphasis on "dependent" (McLoughlin 1993).

The Supreme Court's decision in the Cherokee Nation case demonstrates significant contradictions within both states' rights and nationalist arguments (Wald 1992). Essentially, the Court upheld the state's integrity against the coexistence of sovereign governments within shared boundaries. The Court's decision, as explained by Chief Justice Marshall appeared to turn on the unique "condition of the Indians in relation to the United States [that] is, perhaps, unlike that of any other two people in existence." Ultimately, the case was about the incomprehensible "hole" in the map within the boundary of Georgia. It was, in fact, an increasing Cherokee nationalism and evidence that the Cherokee planned to remain indefinitely in possession of disputed territory that precipitated Georgia's controversial 1830 legislation.

This decision, however, was reversed the following year in *Worcester v. Georgia.* Under an 1830 law, Georgia required all white residents in Cherokee country to secure a license from the governor and to take an oath of allegiance to the state. Missionaries Samuel A. Worcester and Elizur Butler refused and were convicted and imprisoned. Worcester appealed to the Supreme Court. This time the court found that Indian nations possessed the right under the Constitution, the supreme law of the land, to enter into treaties; that the federal government had exclusive jurisdiction within the boundaries of the Cherokee Nation; and that state law had no force within the Cherokee boundaries. Worcester was ordered released from jail, but President Jackson refused to enforce the court's decision saying: "John Marshall has made his decision, now let him enforce it."

Thus, even though the Cherokee people had adopted many practices of the European settlers and had used the court system in two major Supreme Court cases, they were unable to halt the removal process. The "Americanized" Cherokee evoked anxious responses in their neighbors. This is typified by a statement from the director of the Office of Indian Affairs at the time, Thomas L. McKenney: "They seek to be a People . . . It is much to be regretted that the idea of Sovereignty should have taken such a deep hold of these people" (Wald 1992). Thus, the period of prosperity in the eastern homelands was short and ended rapidly for the Cherokee. The state of Georgia continued to encroach on Indian lands.

In 1835, a small group of Cherokees known as the Treaty Party began negotiating with the federal government. The group, which had no official standing within the Nation, was led by Major Ridge and included his son John, Elias Boudinot (who had established the *Cherokee Phoenix,* America's fist Indian newspaper, in 1828), and Elias's brother, Stand Watie. This group, known as the Ridge Party, signed a treaty at New Echota, Georgia, in 1835. In the treaty, the Ridge Party agreed to sell their eastern homelands for $5 million and to move beyond the Mississippi River to Indian Territory. The treaty was negotiated and signed over the protestations of Principal Chief John Ross, who was in Washington, D.C., at the time of the signing. The Treaty of New Echota, named after the capital city of the Cherokee Nation in Georgia, was ratified in Congress by a single vote, despite knowledge that only a minority of Cherokees had accepted it. The Treaty stipulated that within two years the Principal People were to move from their ancestral homeland.

To the end, the Cherokee attempted to uphold the sovereignty of the original Cherokee Nation through the legal system (Starr 1921). For example, the Rattlesnake Springs (Tennessee) Resolution in 1838 sought to establish the inherent sovereignty of the Nation, together with its constitution and laws. At this time, Rattlesnake Springs, located on the north side of the present Cleveland, Tennessee, was the last Federal concentration camp for the Cherokee prior to the Final Removal. The Cherokee's last resolution emerged from the National Committee and Cherokee Council housed in the Aquohee Camp located here. It stated, in part,

> that the whole Cherokee territory, as described in the first article of the treaty of 1819 between the United States and the Cherokee Nation, and, also, in the constitution of the Cherokee Nation, still remains the rightful and undoubted property of the said Cherokee Nation; and that all the damages and losses, direct or indirect, resulting from the enforcement of the alleged stipulations of the pretended treaty of New Echota, are in justice and equity, chargeable to the account of the United States.

It also stated that the Cherokee people "[did] not intend that it shall be so construed as yielding or giving sanction or approval to the pretended treaty of 1835." Among the signers of the resolution were Richard Taylor, President of the National Committee, and Going Snake, Speaker of the Council.

The attempt was futile, however, and the Cherokee were forcibly removed to the Indian Territory west of the Mississippi in the great Indian Removal of 1838–39 (Fogelson and Kutche 1961). President Martin Van Buren ordered the implementation of the Treaty of New Echota in 1838, and U.S. Army troops under the command of Gen. Winfield Scott began rounding up the Cherokees and moving them into stockades in North Carolina, Georgia, Alabama, and Tennessee. The history of the Removal is the history of increased oppression and suffering of the Cherokee people (as well as the Creek, Choctaw, Chickasaw, and Seminole) by state and federal governments under a series of acts and treaties dating from as early as 1802 (Foreman 1966). Gold had been discovered in Georgia even as Europeans sought new lands, and the emerging overlords of the cotton kingdom looked upon the Indian cornfields and saw the potential for plantation cotton. States passed laws to seize Cherokee farmlands, plantations, and homes.

THE REMOVALS

And so, the Native Americans left. First the Choctaw moved out of Mississippi, during a winter blizzard, barefoot and short on blankets and rations. Next the Creek were moved from Alabama, some in chains. They were followed by the Chickasaw from Arkansas and Mississippi, and the Seminole from Florida. And then it was exile time for the Cherokee. They had successfully argued their case before the U.S. Supreme Court and had heard Chief Justice John Marshall affirm their sovereign status and their right to remain in Georgia. However, they found themselves rounded up by President Jackson's soldiers, incarcerated in detention camps, and marched 800 circuitous miles to eastern Indian Territory.

In spite of the increasing pressure to emigrate, only about 2,000 of the eastern Cherokee had been removed by May 23, 1838, the expiration of the time fixed for their departure. Some 15,000 remained (Foreman 1966, 286). Gen. Winfield Scott established his headquarters at New Echota and issued a proclamation that all Cherokee must emigrate at once. He directed the final gathering and removal of the Cherokee people.

Perhaps the magnitude of the event is best captured in the observation of a Georgia volunteer, afterward a Colonel in the Confederate army. "I fought through the Civil War and have seen men shot to pieces and slaughtered by thousands, but the Cherokee removal was the cruelest work I ever knew" (Foreman 1966).

An estimated several hundred to one thousand Cherokee escaped the Removal by hiding in the mountains. They were separated from the political and spiritual leadership of the Nation when the most highly esteemed leaders, guardians of traditional beliefs, joined the approximately 18,000 who emigrated west. Following disastrous relocations by military-supervised river transport, Principal Chief John Ross negotiated with Gen. Winfield Scott to permit the Cherokee to conduct their own removal overland.

Beginning in August 1838, the remaining detainees set out in some thirteen traveling parties. In the fall and early winter of 1838 the last segment of the Cherokee Nation headed overland and by water to the

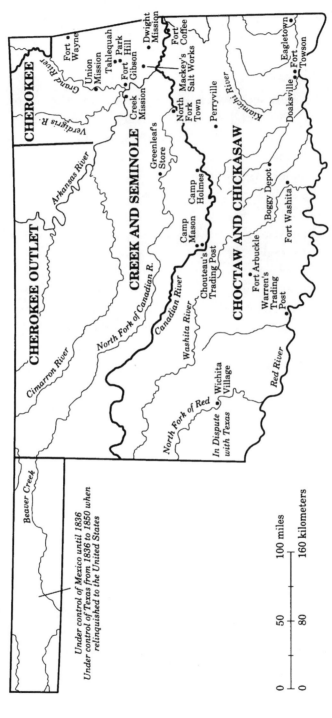

Indian Territory, 1830–1855. Map reprinted, by permission, from Baird and Goble, *The Story of Oklahoma*, © 1994 by the University of Oklahoma Press.

Indian Territory (Figure 1). The Cherokees were separated into contingents of varying size and faced ordeals that ranged from dysentery to hypothermia, from measles to whooping cough. It is estimated that of the total 18,000 Cherokees gathered up to emigrate west after the Treaty of 1835, between 4,000 and 8,000 perished in stockades prior to removal or on the journey to the Indian Territory lands west of the Mississippi (Woodward 1963). The final Cherokee migration was marked by a trail of graves. It became known as the "The Trail Where They Cried" or the "Trail of Tears" (Woodward 1963; Waldman 1985). The expression now stands for the forced removals and suffering of all the Five Tribes (Waldman 1985).

Three detachments of Cherokees, totaling about 2,800 people, traveled by river to Indian Territory. The first left on June 6 by steamboat and barge from Ross' Landing (present-day Chattanooga) on the Tennessee River. They followed the Tennessee River as it wound across northern Alabama. The trip included a short railroad detour around the shoals between Decatur and Tuscumbia Landing. The route then headed north through central Tennessee and Kentucky to the Ohio River. The Ohio took them to the Mississippi, which they followed to the mouth of the Arkansas River. The Arkansas led northwest to Indian Territory, and they arrived aboard a steamboat at the mouth of Sallisaw Creek near Fort Coffee on June 19, 1838. The first groups were the more fortunate. The later two groups suffered from drought and disease (especially the children), and they did not arrive in Indian Territory until the end of the summer. All three groups were more fortunate, however, than the remaining Principal People, who traveled overland to Indian Territory on existing roads.

The overland travelers were organized into detachments ranging in size from 700 to 1,600, with each detachment headed by a "conductor" and an "assistant conductor" appointed by John Ross. The Cherokees who had signed the treaty of New Echota were moved in a separate detachment conducted by a John Bell and administered by U.S. Army Lt. Edward Deas. A physician, and perhaps a clergyman, usually accompanied each detachment. Supplies of flour and corn, and occasionally salt pork, coffee, and sugar were obtained in advance, but were generally of poor quality. Drought and the number of people being moved reduced forage for draft animals, which often were used to haul possessions while the people routinely walked.

The most commonly used overland route followed a northern path, but other detachments followed a variety of more southern routes. The northern route started at Rattlesnake Springs, Tennessee, and crossed central Tennessee, southwestern Kentucky, and southern Illinois. After crossing the Mississippi River north of Cape Girardeau, Missouri, these particular detachments trekked across southern Missouri and the northwest corner of Arkansas. Death was a daily occurrence due to road conditions, illness, and the distresses of winter, particularly in southern Illinois as the people waited to cross the ice-choked Mississippi.

A witness of the entire process observed:

> I saw the helpless Cherokees arrested and dragged from their homes, and driven at the bayonet point into the stockades. [During the hot summer in the stockade, many Cherokee died due to the lack of clean water and proper waste treatment facilities.] And in the chill of a drizzling rain on an October morning I saw them loaded like cattle or sheep into six hundred and forty-five wagons and started toward the west. . . . On the morning of November the 17th we encountered a terrific sleet and snowstorm with freezing temperatures and from that day until we reached the end of the fateful journey on March 26, 1839, the sufferings of the Cherokees were awful. The trail of exiles was a trail of death. They had to sleep in the wagons and on the ground without fire. And I have known as many as twenty-two of them to die in one night of pneumonia due to ill treatment, cold and exposure.
>
> (BURNETT 1839)

Most of the land route detachments entered present-day Oklahoma near Westville and were met by a contingent of U.S. Troops from Fort Gibson on the Arkansas River. The army officially received the Cherokees, who generally went to live with those who had already arrived or awaited land assignments while camped along the Illinois River and its tributaries east of present-day Tahlequah.

ENCROACHMENT ON INDIAN TERRITORY

In the 1820s it was thought that the formation of an extensive Indian colonization zone in the wilderness area west of the Mississippi would stop, once and for all, the clash of cultures over territory and land. By 1825, new Indian lands had been delineated, which in the 1830 came to be called the Indian Territory. In 1834 the Trade and Intercourse Act gave the federal government the right to quarantine Indians there for the purpose of civilizing, or better, "detribalizing" them. At its largest size, in the years before 1854, the Indian Territory extended from the Red River to the Missouri, and from the state lines of Arkansas, Missouri, and Iowa to the 100th meridian, the western boundary of the United States at that time (Waldman 1985).

In the years between the Trail of Tears (1838–39) and the American Civil War (1861–65), the Cherokee Nation once again established itself in pursuits for which the tribe had been noted earlier. The Cherokee accepted the world in which they found themselves. They were diligent in the quest for better education, and demonstrated enlightened stability in government and tribal functions (Tracey 1996). "Renewal" seemed to be a firm and constant philosophical tenet of the Cherokee. On their new lands, as they had done in their eastern homelands, they took advantage of their environment, and many of them once again acquired fine houses and good stock and developed productive fruit orchards.

The name Indian Territory is misleading, for the area never possessed an integrated territorial government. There was, rather, a collection of independent tribal governments. Of course, there was no uniformity in lifestyle since the Indians had come from different regions. Homogeneity and stability were further impeded by the steady flow of white settlers moving westward along the Santa Fe, Oregon, and Mormon trails.

Thus it was in the Territory that the major migration of Cherokee joined the approximately 2,000 Cherokees who had emigrated earlier, between 1836 and 1838, the "Old Settlers" or "Cherokees West," in what is today eastern Oklahoma (Woodward 1963, 195). The new arrivals constituted four-fifths of the Cherokee Nation West.

Friction between the two Cherokee nations emerged. The newly arrived Eastern Cherokees wanted to perpetuate their form of government, but the Western Cherokees expected the easterners to live under their government. The Cherokee who had moved west prior to 1820 lacked a written constitution, had few written laws and paid small heed to education. In addition, traditional religion did not play an important role in their lives.

Again, the promised and presumed inviolate boundaries of the Indian Territory were broached and the Territory under Indian control began to shrink in the 1850s. In the northern section, the most impoverished and disorganized Indians were persuaded to sign away their tribal rights. Subsequently, in 1854 this portion of the Territory became the Kansas and Nebraska territories. In 1862, the Homestead Act opened up Indian lands in the territories to white homesteaders. These settlers were deeded 160-acre plots after living on them for five years.

In the remaining Territory, a further attack on the communal living pattern of the Indians took place in 1887. In that year the U.S. Congress passed the General Allotment Act (called the Dawes' Severalty Act after its sponsor Senator Henry Dawes of Massachusetts), under which reservation land was to be divided into 40 to 160-acre parcels and allotted to heads of Indian families—ostensibly to provide economic motivation for farming and development. Any land remaining after all the "eligibles" had received their shares would be sold to whites. The money from such sales would be used to pay for Indian schooling. However, the Cherokee and Choctaw refused allotment. After all, the Cherokee already had schools.

In response, in 1891 legislation was passed that provided for leasing of the allotted lands to whites. In fact, the Cherokee were forced to sell, for roughly $1.40 an acre, the Cherokee Outlet, originally an eight-million-acre swath of land extending from the (then) edge of the Nation some two hundred miles west into the High Plains. The Outlet had been set aside to guarantee that the tribe would have unobstructed access for hunting buffalo. But the buffalo had been slaughtered, and white homesteaders were massing along the border of the Outlet for what some Oklahomans still proudly claim as "the greatest land rush in the history of the American West" (Norman 1995).

> For among the arrival of waves of white settlers in the early 1800s were trappers and traders who made their living selling meat and hides. By the 1870s, hundreds of thousands of buffalo hides, tongues and bones (ground up for use as phosphorous fertilizer) were shipped eastward each year. During the winter of 1872–73 an estimated 1.5 million were shipped aboard trains and wagons. Some U.S. government officials reportedly promoted the destruction of

the bison herds as a way to weaken American Indians in the region. Congressman James Throckmorton of Texas believed that "it would be a great step forward in the civilization of the Indians and preservation of peace on the border if there was not a buffalo in existence."

NATURE PROGRAM, "AMERICAN BUFFALO: SPIRIT OF A NATION."
See http://www.pbs.org/wnet/nature/buffalo/nation.html

Another congressional act in 1893 empowered the Dawes Commission to deal individually with each of the Five Tribes. Included among the tribes so designated were the Cherokee, Creek, Choctaw, Chickasaw, and Seminole. These tribes held millions of acres of land in the Cotton Belt and were known as the most civilized tribes in America. They had adopted the agricultural system of their white neighbors, including the institution of black chattel slavery. The Act of 1893 empowered the federal government to procure agreements for allotment of lands in severalty and to lay the groundwork for the subsequent dissolution of tribal governments, preparatory to Oklahoma statehood. And, in a final move to destroy tribal life of the Cherokee and Choctaw, Congress passed the Curtis Act of 1898, which dissolved the Cherokee and Choctaw tribal governments and unilaterally extended the land allotment policy to them (Waldman 1985). The Cherokee Nation was dissolved at the time of Oklahoma statehood in 1907.

Thus, upon the arrival of the twentieth century, the Cherokee were subject to federal and state policies that effectively sought to eliminate tribal land holdings and political organizations, and to suppress or destroy communal customs. Acculturation was enforced also by laws requiring the cutting of traditionally long hair and the outlawing of cultural rituals such as dance. At the same time, federally administered schools sought to educate Native Americans in the social customs of white society.

The final blow came with the admission of Oklahoma to the Union in 1907. Prior to this, the Cherokee government was to have been dissolved by March 1906. However, it was continued in a modified and restricted form under an act of Congress until June 1914. Although the majority of Cherokee became citizens of the newly formed State, subject to its laws, full-blood Keetoowahs retreated to the more remote sections of eastern Oklahoma, where they sought to maintain ancient tribal traditions (Woodward 1963).

The result of these policies as well as the general development of cities led to considerable Indian urbanization. In fact, the rate of farm-to-city migration by Native Americans before the 1930s was roughly the same as for the whole U.S. population at comparable levels of industrialization. An investigation of conditions on reservations and a critique of federal Indian policy was begun in 1924 and published in 1928, known as the Meriam Report. The survey was conducted in gratitude for the Indians' services to the country in World War I. The report documented shocking conditions on the reservations, predicted continued urbanization, and urged the government to help Indians in making the transition (Meriam 1928).

At the federal level, a Division of Medical Assistance was created within the Bureau of Indian Affairs in 1910. This evolved into the Division of Indian Health in 1924. Three years earlier, the Snyder Act of 1921 had given responsibility for Native American social, educational, and medical services to the Department of the Interior.

REVERSALS

Under the impetus of the Meriam Report, findings documenting the Indians' general failure to adopt and/or adapt to the majority culture in the urban environment, once again caused the focus of government intervention to change. In the 1930s John Collier, the Commissioner of Indian Affairs, promoted a kind of cultural and political pluralism that sought to end the long-standing policy of forced assimilation. His proposed Indian Reorganization Act was passed by Congress, allowing tribes to retain some degree of sovereignty and to develop as much as possible within the contexts of their own cultures (Burt 1986). In 1934, acknowledging the failure of past policies of forced acculturation, Congress passed the Indian Reorganization Act to reverse the policies of assimilation and allotment. Tribal land holdings were given legal sanction, unsold allotted lands were returned to the tribes, funds for the purchase of new lands were provided, and tribal constitutions were encouraged, as were tribal systems of justice and business corporations.

By 1945, however, several bills to abolish Native American reservations were introduced; relocation changed in both purpose and provision in the three decades following World War II. During the 1950s once again the federal government would approach Native Americans with a renewed coercive "assimilationist" policy. "Termination" (of Indian cultural identity) became the catch phrase that described the assumptions and ideas behind the change in federal Indian policy (Burt 1986).

Broadly interpreted, it meant integrating Native Americans into the mainstream legally, socially, and economically as a means to diminish the federal role in Indian affairs and to end support for services provided to Native Americans. More specifically, however, termination referred to a process of tribe-by-tribe legislation, revoking the tribal charters that under Collier's Indian Reorganization Act had stood as the foundation for Indian sovereignty and Indian status as distinct peoples within American society. Indian sovereignty and "dual citizenship" were now deemed unacceptable and the traditional Indian communal social structures were perceived to be in conflict with the individualism of the United States.

The Indian Citizenship Act of 1924 granted U.S. citizenship to all Native Americans. It was argued, therefore, that the government should deal with Indians as individuals rather than as members of discrete social and political groups. Separate Indian governments and related property rights, dependency on services supplied by the federal government, and the continued existence of the Bureau of Indian Affairs itself was viewed as a violation of a politico-economic system based upon individual property rights and private enterprise. A majority opinion held that Indians should be freed from government paternalism in order to enjoy the freedoms derived from competition as individuals within the marketplace (Burt 1986).

Acts and laws were passed establishing funding for "voluntary" relocation programs. The BIA worked out cooperative arrangements with the United States Employment Service to assist Indians in finding jobs in cities. Moving Native Americans into the cities was much less expensive and involved a smaller federal role than other options such as improving the health and economic status of persons living on reservations. In 1952, under Commissioner Dillon Myer, Operation Relocation began and the first permanent migrants from a number of tribes began moving to cities. Also spurring relocation was removal of tribal civil and criminal jurisdiction on reservations. Therefore, for many, the decision to relocate was not based on the positive attraction provided by economic opportunities of the city but rather on an increasingly negative situation on the reservations, fostered at least in part by decreased federal funding for remedial programs.

The Indian Health Service (IHS) was established in 1955 within the Department of Health, Education and Welfare (now Health and Human Services). The mission of the IHS was to raise the level of health among Indians to the highest possible level, later interpreted as the same level of health extant within the general population.

To summarize, the relocation programs intended to remove the Native Americans from the reservations and into the mainstream of life in the U.S. were largely failures. Studies indicate that Indians who stayed in the cities were only marginally more economically prosperous than those remaining on reservations. The most prosperous were those with existing job skills or experience off the reservation. Many migrants became part of a growing underclass of minorities in central cities and large numbers returned or attempted to return to reservations. Relocation also failed to achieve the hoped for cultural assimilation among Native Americans to any great extent. And, somewhat paradoxically, pan-Indian social institutions developed in cities that would eventually serve as the foundation for political activism based on Native American identity. Opposition to the relocation programs increased and culminated in a reversal in 1977, when the American Indian Policy Review Commission opposed forced assimilation of Native Americans and advocated tribal self-determination and self-government.

CHEROKEE NATIONAL GOVERNMENT

During this period of reversals, some members of the Cherokee Tribes pursued a movement to reconstitute the Cherokee National Government. Interestingly, this movement began in the 1950s, the period of renewed assimilationist policies on the part of the federal government.

Today the Cherokee Nation is the second largest Indian tribe in the United States. There are more than 182,000 tribal members, and almost

70,000 Cherokees live within the 7,000 square mile area of the Cherokee Nation—a jurisdictional service area that includes all of eight counties and portions of six counties in northeastern Oklahoma. The jurisdictional area lies within the boundaries of the historical Cherokee Nation, as developed after the Trail of Tears and prior to the Civil War. Most of the Cherokee Nation rests on the Ozark Plateau, a place of spring-fed creeks, riffled rivers, carved valleys, and undulant hills. It stretches from the prairie plains in the north and west to the foothills of the Boston Mountains in the east.

The Nation's capital is Tahlequah, a town of approximately 11,000 in Cherokee County, some 66 miles southeast of Tulsa near the western terminus of the Trail of Tears. Cherokee farmers near the capital grow blueberries, peaches, and soybeans. To promote education and employment, the tribe works closely with a local university and recruits firms to open manufacturing plants in the region. The Cherokee Nation has approximately $115 million in assets, a net worth of approximately $70 million, and an annual budget of approximately $100 million, 62 percent of which comes from the federal government. As a federally recognized Indian tribe, the Cherokee Nation has both the opportunity and the sovereign right to exercise control over and development of tribal assets, which includes 62,000 acres of land, as well as 96 miles of the Arkansas River bed.

The Cherokee Nation has a tripartite democratic form of government, including judicial, executive, and legislative branches. The Commissioner of Indian Affairs on September 5, 1975, approved a revised constitution of the Nation. The Cherokee people ratified it in June of 1976. On February 10, 1990, the Nation completed negotiations with the federal government on a tribal self-governance agreement for direct funding from the U.S. Congres. The agreement authorizes the Nation to plan, conduct, consolidate, and administer programs and to receive direct funding to be used in delivering services to tribal members. Self-governance represents a change from the paternalistic controls that the federal government exercised in the past to the full-tribal autonomy and independence intended by the treaties with sovereign Indian nations.

It was the spirit of survival and perseverance that carried the Cherokee to Indian Territory on the Trail of Tears when the original Cherokee

Nation in the eastern homelands was dissolved. And it was that same spirit that sustained the Cherokee through development and implementation of the "Act of Union" signed in Tahlequah on September 6, 1839, which formally merged the eastern and western Cherokee governments in Oklahoma. This Cherokee Nation was forced to dissolve when Oklahoma became a state in 1907. Undaunted, the Cherokee Nation reestablished. In 1971 the Cherokee Nation's government was reorganized. The mission of the government of the current Cherokee Nation is to "promote and sustain the self-reliance of its members. All programs will strive to develop an individual's independence by enhancing his or her knowledge, skills and self-responsibility. Inherent in this objective is the recognition that needs are best defined and met by individuals and the communities in which they live" (Cherokee Nation 1997). In the chapters that follow, several important strategies the Nation uses to fulfill its mission will be described and related to major challenges faced in the development and delivery of health services to its people.

CHAPTER TWO

Implications of Indian Identification for Health Care Eligibility

This chapter focuses on the continuing and increasingly complex issue of Indian identification and on questions pertaining to their eligibility for federal government health services. The goal here is to examine the question of Native American eligibility for such services, thereby providing insight into an issue that is likely to reappear as the pressure to contain the costs of health and social programs continues and even escalates. When the rights of any minority groups are challenged, it is particularly important to examine the issue carefully and to provide relevant documentation. The focus in this chapter, to that end, is directed toward five related issues and questions:

Definition of eligibility: Who is a Native American or on what basis is one defined as Native American?

Appropriate authority: Who has the legitimate and ultimate authority to make a determination of identity and, hence, eligibility?

Cherokee identity: What criteria do the Cherokee employ to determine identity?

Eligibility criteria: On what eligibility criteria do Natives receive direct service benefits from the Indian Health Service?

Potential effects: What is the potential impact on health care of changes in the federal government's definitions of Native Americans?

The discussion begins with an overview of the Indian population in North America and the United States. This is followed by a historical review of constitutional issues surrounding the broader questions of the status of Native Americas and the potential long-term impact of proposed changes in the regulations governing eligibility for Indian Health Service benefits. Providing complete answers would require legal, constitutional, and ethical research beyond the scope of this chapter. Therefore, a brief account of the nature and evolution of the federal-Indian relationship is presented here, along with a description of criteria used in the definition and identification of Native Americans for the purpose of receiving health care benefits from the Indian Health Service. And perhaps most importantly, this chapter will discuss some of the long-term implications of policy changes related to changes in the definition of eligibility for health services by the Department of Health and Human Services.

SOME BASIC QUESTIONS

The actual number of Indians in North America in the past as well as in the present remains a conundrum. Throughout the years, people from a number of walks of life and varying levels of expertise have provided estimates. For example, in 1841, George Catlin (1796-1872), the artist who specialized in painting American Indian scenes, published a two-volume work entitled *Letters and Notes on the Manners, Customs, and Condition of the North American Indians.* Based upon his extensive travels among Native Americans, he estimated the number of Indians in North America in 1492 to be 16 million. In 1860 the missionary Emmanuel Domenech concurred, estimating the population to have been between 16 and 17 million. In 1924, however, the geographer Karl Sapper placed the total Indian population in 1492 at between 2.5 million and 3.5 million.

The range in estimates has not diminished substantially as recent history textbooks place the Indian population of North America in 1492 anywhere from 1 million to 12 million (Daniels 1992). More than a century of debate has produced no generally accepted population estimates and no consensus on the methods of developing them. This lack of agreement reflects both the diverse conclusions of experts and the inadequacy of historical evidence.

To the best of our knowledge, none of the Indians living in what are now the United States and Canada kept written records, and what records they did keep did not contain population counts. Researchers must make do with invariably defective reports and accounts by contemporary European explorers, soldiers, traders, and priests. To date at least, accuracy in estimating the number of Indians in North America is impossible to achieve for the earliest period of European contact. Whether the actual number is 2 million, 5 million, or 16 million, the number of North American Indians had declined to fewer than 250,000 by the end of the nineteenth century.

As recorded in the U.S. Census, however, since 1900 there has been a steady increase in the American Indian population. In 1980 some 7.1 million Americans listed an Indian ancestry, although only 1.36 million reported their race to be Indian (Snipp 1989). In 1990 the U.S. Census recorded a total of just fewer than 2 million American Indians, Eskimos, or Aleuts identified by race (U.S. Bureau of the Census 1993). In addition to the increase in Indians among the general population, the number of Native Americans and Alaska Native service populations in Indian Health Services Areas (IHS Areas) continues to increase. According to the 1990 U.S. Census, there were 1,207,236 Native Americans living within the twelve IHS Areas. In 1998, according to the Census estimates, a total of 1,462,578 Indians were residing in these Areas (IHS 1994). The Oklahoma Service Area containing the Cherokee Nation had a 1990 population of 262,517 and an estimated 1998 population of 303,404. This particular service area has the largest population of any IHS Area.

Despite the "authority" attributed by some to the U.S. Census figures, there remains considerable confusion as to the true population figures. The increased Indian population can be attributed, in part, to a relatively high birth rate among Indians and Alaska Natives. The estimated crude birth rate (births per 1,000 population) among this population for the period 1989-91 was 28.1 compared to a rate of about 16.5 for all races in the United States. Nevertheless, the 1989-91 crude birth rate among Indians and Alaska Natives reflects a rather steady decrease from the 1972-74 rate of 31.7. During this same period, the crude birth rate for all races in the United States increased rather steadily from a 1972 rate of 14.8 (IHS 1994).

WHAT IS AN INDIAN?

During debate on the annual Indian appropriation bill on February 24, 1896, the question "What is an Indian?" emerged. At that time, Congressman Charles Curtis of Kansas proposed those mixed-blood children of white men and Indian women should have "the same right and privileges to the property and annuities of the tribe to which the mother belongs, by blood, as any other member of the tribe." Interior Secretary Hoke Smith had only recently denied those rights, based upon his interpretation of an 1888 federal statute barring non-Indian husbands from acquiring a legal right to the property of their Indian wives. Curtis' proposal was not altogether altruistic as he argued that "mixed-blood" was a powerful instrument in the government's assimilation program. "We may talk all we please; missionaries may say what they please," said Curtis; "but the only way to solve the Indian question is by education and by intermarriage of Indians and whites" (Record 1896).

Curtis was not alone in the debate regarding Indian identity in the 1890s. Earlier, Indian Commissioner Thomas Jefferson Morgan, in his 1892 annual report to Congress, submitted an analysis of the problem that dated back to the arrival of Columbus in 1492. He noted that the federal government had passed many laws "without discriminating as to those over whom it has a right to exercise such control." If mixed-bloods were not Indians, then it was a serious question as to whether "real Indians" might not have an equitable claim against the government for the misappropriation of their annuities.

Careful students of mid-nineteenth-century Indian demography were obliged to conclude that while the full-blood population was declining dramatically, the opposite was true of the mixed-bloods (Unrau 1989). Today, the issue of identity further confuses the situation with regard to the number of Indians. While some of the growth in the Indian and Alaska Native population derives from a natural increase, perhaps the largest percentage of the population growth can be attributed to increased personal identification. This has resulted from a changing awareness and increased self-esteem among people of Native American ancestry, a phenomenon referred to by some authors as "resurgent ethnicity" or "ethnogenesis" (Nagel 1996). A demographic analysis of the 1980 census statistics concluded, for example, that much of the growth in the

Indian population was the result of "new identifications": "reporting of an 'Indian' census race by Americans of varying degrees of Indian ancestry who formerly reported a non-Indian race" in earlier censuses (Eschbach 1992).

Not only has the Indian population increased rapidly due to this resurgent ethnicity, but it has become more dispersed as well. In 1930, for example, almost 80 percent of Native Americans and Alaska Natives lived in nine states and in the territory of Alaska (Eschbach 1992). By 1990, however, only about 50 percent of Indians lived in these (now) ten states. In nine western states, the Indian population rose from 14 to 24 percent of the total number. And in the eastern half of the country, the Indian population rose from 9 to 27 percent of the general population in the region.

An analysis of the cause of this national dispersal determined that it was overwhelmingly the result of new identifications as Indian rather than actual migration from old Indian areas. For example, in 1990, Indian parents reported more than half of their children born in California who were between ages ten and nineteen in 1980 as belonging to some other race (Eschbach 1992). Similarly, in eastern states almost 80 percent of the Indians who were between the ages of twenty and twenty-nine in 1960 were not identified as Indians by their parents in 1960.

On the other hand, traditional Indian areas also had "over count" ratios. Among the highest of these areas was Oklahoma. This finding was not surprising due to the reported confusion of Indian ethnic boundaries in the state, where 59 percent of marriages by Indians in 1980 were to non-Indians. Nevertheless, almost all of the apparent geographic redistribution of the Indian population between prior censuses and the 1980 census was attributed to changes in identification rather than to migration. Significant proportions of the Indian population native to eastern regions, and in California in the west, were enumerated in previous censuses as some non-Indian race, even in the self-identification censuses in 1960 and 1970.

The questions of race and ethnicity are not new to Native Americans generally, or to the Cherokee specifically. In their early struggle for independence, the Cherokee honored their own stories of indigenous racial origin. However, after 1794 when they made their first peace with the

Euro-Americans, they were compelled to react to efforts to impose concepts of "race difference" upon them (McLoughlin and Conser 1989).

In an effort to assert their own ethnic dignity and identity, and reflecting an accretion of the religious teaching of missionaries and early European contacts, the Cherokee full bloods frankly asserted that they were the first people created by the Great Spirit and were always his favorite. And further, they would remain his chosen people as long as they adhered to his will and spiritual laws. Indeed, early missionaries reported that some of the more important Cherokee post-contact religious mythology could be traced to biblical stories. As early as 1820, a Cherokee shaman reportedly told a missionary that the white people had borrowed stories from the Cherokee to put in their "good book" (Washburn 1869). In any event, from the Cherokee perspective, to be or become an American would require a pluralistic concept of ethnicity, for the United States would always be a multiracial nation.

In the increasingly pluralistic and ethnically complex U.S. society, questions frequently are raised concerning racial/ethnic identity and race classification. This is manifest, for example, in a move to add a "mixed race" self-identification to the 2000 U.S. Census. Although it is an attempt at reflecting the increased integration of society over the past several decades, this move is being opposed by some members of racial minorities. The opposition derives from the presumed potential negative impact of reduced federal funding for population-programs targeted to them should their populations be decreased by inclusion of the new category.

The current debate demonstrates the importance and at the same time the difficulty of determining the "race" of any individual. Is a racial category strictly biological, or is it to be determined by a combination of biology, culture, and social integration? Or should race be determined simply on the basis of self-identification? On what basis should an individual be classified a member of a group that is eligible for federal assistance?

Questions such as these have been important to Native Americans for a considerable time. Native Americans are geographically dispersed, linguistically diverse, and culturally varied. Nevertheless, few researchers would deny that there is at least some commonality and validity to the category "American Indian," or "Native American." On the one hand, this common identification is assumed and promulgated in federal law. Federal Indian law resides in a special volume of the United States Code. American Indians are the only ethnic group with whom treaties were made and whose special status was acknowledged in the U.S. Constitution (Nagel 1996).

Questions about who should be eligible for the federal government's health services for Native Americans have been raised periodically over the past century, for example in the 1950s when the Bureau of Indian Affairs (BIA) adopted a policy of assimilating Native Americans into mainstream American life (Fuchs 1974). This was to be accomplished by providing funding for relocating them into urban areas and, wherever possible, providing them initial employment. As one senator commented at the time: "the sooner we can get the Indians into the cities, the sooner the government can get out of Indian business" (Bahr, et al. 1972).

The policy of "urbanizing" Native Americans as implemented by the BIA was unsuccessful. Many Indians remained on reservations, and urban areas proved to an inhospitable environment for many of those who migrated. At the outset, Indians viewed the BIA policy and decisions with considerable apprehension. A major source of dissatisfaction with the BIA was the lack of genuine Indian involvement in its policy decisions (Bashshur 1979). Native Americans who did move to urban areas were confronted with economic difficulties and the same kinds of discrimination encountered there by other minority groups (Jorgensen 1971). Nevertheless, the "removal" programs of the BIA, coupled with promises of attractive financial settlements for their lands, prompted tribes such as the Klamath in Oregon and the Penobscot in Maine to terminate formal relationships with the federal government. Subsequently, both of these tribes found it necessary to spend considerable time, effort, and money to get reinstated during the 1960s and 1970s.

Again, however, in the early 1980s, with the increasing numbers of people identifying themselves as Native Americans, the relationship between the federal government and Indian tribes was at issue. Perhaps fueled by the rising program costs associated with the rising numbers of Indians, the question this time pondered who should be eligible for federally sponsored programs rather than a termination of government-to-government relationships. The efforts to redefine eligibility focused on the Native programs sponsored by the Department of Health and Human Services and the Department of the Interior. Some Native Americans viewed the federal government's efforts as an attempt to deny benefits to them. Federal officials, meanwhile, were being driven by the rapidly rising costs of these as well as other health care programs.

In 1997 news reports indicated that the status of the American Indian tribes was again under question. With little debate and no public hearings, a Senate subcommittee approved two measures that would have removed some of the oldest principles in how the nation's 554 tribes are governed and would have deprived them of basic operating money if they did not agree to the changes. The sponsor of the measure hoped to force a significant change in the long-standing status that tribes have had as nations within a nation (Times 8/27/97). The reported strategy is to gain support for the measures from the senators of 17 states without federally recognized Indian tribes.

THE FEDERAL-INDIAN RELATIONSHIP

The relationship between Native Americans and the U.S. federal government is complex, and it presents a unique set of problems that do not lend themselves to easy comprehension or resolution. That is why it is understandable that a majority of the American public may fail to recognize or appreciate these complexities. In addition, some seventeen states do not currently have federally recognized Indian tribes residing in them. So, for many Americans, problems pertaining to Native Americans are the problems of "other states." Generally, when non-Native Americans, including many in government, do consider the situation of Native Americans vis-à-vis the federal government, they tend to place the relationships under the umbrella of "treaty obligations." It would seem that this attitude has permeated the thinking and contributed to the posture of even some federal officials responsible for Native American affairs. It is not certain that the nature of these obligations is fully appreciated even at such levels.

United States constitutional law concerning Native American tribes and individuals is unique and separate from the rest of American jurisprudence. Nonetheless, when discussing Indian law it is common for individuals to refer to general constitutional law, civil rights law, and public land law. This is both erroneous and misleading. Indian law encompasses Western European international law, specific provisions of the U.S. Constitution, pre-colonial treaties, treaties with the United States, a separate and entire volume of the United States Code, as well as numerous decisions of the U.S. Supreme Court and lower federal courts (U.S. Civil Rights Commission 1981).

Several legal concepts have become fundamental to the definition of the relationship between the federal government and Native Americans. Two of these will be addressed here, namely: (1) Native American tribes are governmental units that have a special political relationship with the government of the United States; and (2) Congress is viewed in American jurisprudence as possessing plenary power with respect to Native American affairs, that is, full, complete and unqualified.

Native Americans have long respected and participated in the American process of pursuing legal remedies to questions of conflict between themselves and various governmental entities, including counties, states, and the federal government. They have resorted to the judicial system repeatedly since the early days of the Unites States in attempts to resolve pending legal and/or political disputes. The analytical framework upon which Indian law rests was established by the U.S. Supreme Court over 160 years ago in the *Cherokee Nation v. Georgia*, 30 U.S. 1 (1831).

Briefly, this case involved the state of Georgia and the Cherokees who resided on land that Georgia claimed under its jurisdiction. Beginning in 1791, a series of treaties between the United States and the Cherokees living in Georgia gave recognition to the Cherokees as a nation with their own laws and customs. Nevertheless, subsequent treaties and agreements gradually whittled away at this territory. The issue of states' rights and a prolonged dispute between Georgia and the federal government further complicated the Cherokee situation. In 1802 Georgia was the last of the original colonies to cede its western lands to the federal government. In so doing, Georgia expected all titles to the land held by Indians to be extinguished. However, that did not happen, and the Cherokee continued to occupy their traditional homelands, which had been guaranteed to them by treaty: "Inclination to remove from this land has no abiding place in our hearts, and when we move we shall move by the course of nature to sleep under this ground which the Great Spirit gave to our ancestors and which now covers them in their undisturbed peace" (Young 1996).

Despite the fact that it had explicitly transferred all its legal authority with respect to Native Americans to the federal government when it ratified the Constitution, the state of Georgia continued to impose its state laws on the Cherokee who resided within the Nation's self-declared boundaries (Prucha 1981). Settlers continued to encroach on Cherokee lands, as well as lands belonging to the neighboring Creek Indians. In 1828 Georgia passed a law pronouncing all laws of the Cherokee Nation to be null and void after June 1, 1830, forcing a dispute with the federal government over the issue of states' rights. Georgia no longer recognized the rights of the Cherokee Nation and passed a law declaring it illegal for Cherokees "to gather and meet in groups of three or more" (Prucha 1981). Tribal meetings had to be held just across the state boundary line at Red Clay, Tennessee. When gold was discovered on Cherokee land in northern Georgia in 1829, efforts to dislodge the Cherokees from their lands intensified.

At about the same time, in 1830, Congress passed the Indian Removal Act, which directed the executive branch to negotiate for Indian lands. This act, in combination with the discovery of gold and an increasingly untenable position with the state of Georgia, prompted the Cherokee Nation to bring suit in the U.S. Supreme Court. The suit was filed under Article III of the Constitution. The article gives the Supreme Court original jurisdiction in cases and controversies involving states and foreign nations. The key issue on which the Court was asked to rule was whether the "Cherokees constitute a foreign nation in the sense of the Constitution." In *Cherokee Nation v. Georgia* (1831), Chief Justice John Marshall, writing for the majority, held that the Cherokee Nation was a "domestic dependent nation," and, therefore, Georgia state law applied to them.

The concept of "domestic dependent nation" introduced by the Supreme Court was significant in at least two ways. First, it acknowledged the governmental status of tribes, albeit domestic, and it affirmed their special, dependent relationship. Chief Justice John Marshall explained the nature of the political relationship of tribes to the federal government and characterized it as that of a trust, "a ward to a guardian." He further established the basic principles underlying the fiduciary relationship.

That Supreme Court decision, however, was reversed the following year in *Worcester v. Georgia*. Under a law of 1830, which went into effect on February 1, 1831, Georgia required all white residents in Cherokee country to secure a license from the governor and to take an oath of allegiance to the state. It also made it an offense punishable by four years' imprisonment in the penitentiary to refuse to do so. Missionaries Samuel A. Worcester and Elizur Butler refused to sign the oath. They were indicted in the Superior Court of Gwinnett County for residing without license in that part of the Cherokee country attached to Georgia by her laws and in violation of the act of her legislature. They were convicted and imprisoned. Worcester appealed to the Supreme Court. This time the court found that: Indian Nations are capable of making treaties; under the Constitution, treaties are the supreme law of the land; the federal government has exclusive jurisdiction within the boundaries of the Cherokee Nation; and, the state law has no force within the Cherokee boundaries. The legislation of Georgia on the subject was therefore determined to be unconstitutional and void (Royce 1975). Worcester was ordered released from jail.

Nevertheless, three components of the trust relationship evolved: land ownership, tribal self-government, and social service. Though of obvious importance, the first two components are beyond the scope of the present discussion. The focus here is on social services because it includes the trust responsibility to provide health services. The meaning and implications of this component have been debated on frequent occasions, but the view expressed by the American Indian Policy Review Commission (1976) seems to prevail, to wit:

> The purpose behind the trust is and always has been to insure the survival and welfare of Indian tribes and people. This includes those services required to protect and enhance Indian lands, resources and self-government, and also includes those economic and social programs, which are necessary to raise the standard of living and social well being of the Indian people to a level comparable to the non-Indian society. This duty has long been recognized implicitly by Congress in numerous acts, including the Snyder Act of 1921, the Indian Reorganization Act of 1934, the Johnson-O'Malley Act of 1934, the Native American Programs Act of 1974,

the Indian Self-Determination and Education Assistance Act of 1975, and the Indian Health Care Improvement Act of 1976. In fact, as early as 1819, Congress established a general civilization fund to aid Indians in achieving self-sufficiency within the non-Indian social and economic structure.

It is reasonably safe to conclude that the intentions of the Congress were clearly stated here and the laws for governing Native affairs were quite explicit (Office of Technology and Assessment 1986). For instance, it is clear that the power to govern relationships with Native Americans rests with the Congress, whereas the Executive branch has only that power that Congress explicitly authorizes in this regard. People may choose to find fault or disagree with the congressional intent and the laws that pertain to the Federal-Indian relationship, but the interpretations and intent of laws established by the Congress and the Supreme Court have been consistent over the years.

Also, there is little question that Indian law affirms that the U.S. Congress retains plenary power with respect to Indian affairs, as explained earlier. The Constitution declared that the Congress has the power to "regulate commerce with foreign nations and among several states, and with the Indian tribes." This was confirmed by the Supreme Court in its opinion in *United States v. Sandoval*, 231 U.S. 28 (1913): "Not only does the Constitution expressly authorize Congress to regulate commerce with the Indian tribes, but long continued legislative and executive usage and an unbroken current of judicial decisions have attributed to the United States the power and duty of exercising a fostering care and protection over all dependent Indian communities within its borders whether within or without the limits of a State."

Several conclusions can be drawn from this discussion. Among the more notable are the following: (1) Native American tribes do have unique roles and responsibilities in American society by virtue of their special status as "domestic dependent nations." (When people speak about the "special relationship" between the federal government and Indian tribes, this should be the referent concept.) (2) The U.S. Congress has the plenary power to intercede and resolve conflicts regarding policy questions and other forms of dispute that may arise between tribal organizations and the U.S. Government or any of its agencies. (3)

The stated principles governing Federal-Indian relationships have been tested and challenged many times in the past and have been consistently affirmed by the U.S. Supreme Court and the Congress.

DEPENDENCY

In Chief Justice John Marshall's brief and in the conclusions reached above, the concept of dependency is central. Dependency is at once a complex and sensitive subject and the term should be examined in the context of the Federal-Indian relationship. Only a brief mention is made here of differences in interpretation of the concept and the potential for confusion these difference engender. (The topic is addressed at length in a subsequent chapter dealing with the issue of self-help among members of the Cherokee Nation.) In the historical context developed here, it is important to note that dependency may have an automatic negative connotation within a dominant culture that stresses individualism and independence (Gurian 1977). Historically and in many traditional cultures today, however, dependency often is viewed as a positive attribute. This is particularly true among Native Americans currently seeking revitalization and those seeking remedy for alienation.

Indeed, much of the confusion arising in relationships between Native Americans and the federal government may be traced to a different interpretation, characterization, and implementation of dependency. As Native American people have traditionally understood dependency, it was not condemned or infantile; it was a given of life, an important part of natural being. As defined in Euro-American terms, however, dependence is a necessity at infancy, and the healthy personality sheds it as a part of maturation. The difference in interpretation of the dependency concept has colored the attitudes of Euro-Americans and Native Americans. And it has affected relationships between the groups historically and to this day.

The Bureau of Indian Affairs was established within the Department of the Interior and charged with responsibility for "civilizing" the Indians and implementing federal policy. In the minds of some, in carrying out its responsibility the Bureau has acted to suppress Indian culture, tribal governance, Indian languages, religious, and other cultural practices (Josephy 1968).

THE INDIAN HEALTH SERVICE

The responsibility of the United States to Indian tribal governments and their members for the provision of health care was established in numerous treaties with Indian tribes in which the United States agreed to provide such services (Select Committee 1992). For example, in Article 2 of the 1854 treaty with the Rogue River Indians (10 Stat. 1119), the United States agreed that "'provision shall be made'for a hospital, medicines, and a physician." The responsibility has been further delineated and defined by numerous statutes and administrative regulations. Thus, the United States has long assumed a legal and moral obligation to provide adequate health care and services to Indian tribes and their members.

Through the military, the federal government provided health care services to Native Americans as early as the beginning of the nineteenth century. In 1902, for example, U.S. Army doctors worked to cure outbreaks of smallpox among Indians living near military posts. The responsibility for providing health care shifted from the military to the civilian sector of government in 1849 when the Bureau of Indian Affairs transferred the authority from the War Department to the Department of Interior.

In 1921 Indian health appropriations became public law with the enactment of the Snyder Act (25 U.S.C. 13). This Act authorized the Bureau of Indian Affairs to provide a selection of services, including those for "relief of distress and conservation of health." This represented the culmination of the historical provision of services to federally recognized Indians, which grew out of the constitutionally based primacy of Congress over Indian affairs. By 1926 medical officers in the Public Health Service (PHS) were detailed to positions in the Indian Health Program. The Department of Interior under this authorization until 1955 administered Indian health programs. They were then transferred to the Division of Indian Health (now the Indian Health Service) in the Department of Health Education and Welfare (now the U.S. Department of Health and Human Services), pursuant to the Transfer Act (42 U.S.C. 2001).

Thus, it was not until July 1, 1955, that the Indian Health Service was organized within the U.S. Public Health Service. The expressed purpose of the IHS was to raise the level of health among Native Americans "to the highest possible level." Prior to establishment of the IHS, American Indian and Alaska Native affairs fell under the jurisdiction of the Bureau. As one observer commented, "prior to the organization of the IHS, there was no comprehensive health policy for Indians" (Bashshur 1979). The IHS delivers health care to eligible Indians through three different mechanisms. It does so directly through its own facilities, which include hospitals, health centers, school health centers, and smaller health stations; the tribal health delivery system, administered by tribal governments and tribal groups through contracts with IHS these types of facilities as well. Finally, where services are not offered directly through IHS or tribal facilities, limited funds are available in each area for the purchase of care on a contractual basis from non-federal, non-tribal hospitals, clinics, physicians, and dentists.

In response to documented deficiencies in the health status of American Indians and Alaska Natives, the Congress, in 1976, enacted the Indian Health Care Improvement Act (P.L. 94-437). A major purpose of the Act was to improve the health status of American Indians and Alaska Natives, to a level comparable to that of the general population, over a seven-year period or by the end of fiscal year 1984. The Act authorized supplemental funds for Indian healthcare directed toward reducing unmet needs under existing programs and also toward establishing new program efforts, including personnel training and urban health clinics. Because the 1976 Act provided funding for only three years, the Congress revised and extended the authorization in 1980 to cover the period through September 30, 1984 (P.L. 96-537). The Act was again revised and extended in 1988 (P.L. 100-713).

As of October 1993, the IHS and tribes operated a combined total of 49 hospitals (41 IHS, 8 tribal) and 461 outpatient facilities (114 IHS, 347 tribal) across the United States. One hundred percent of all IHS and tribal hospitals as well as 100 percent of all IHS-eligible health centers were accredited as of January 1, 1994. The number of outpatient visits in fiscal year 1993 totaled over 5.5 million, 3.5 million of which were to primary care providers (physicians 2.67 million) (IHS 1994). Based upon 1982-1991 vital events and the 1980 and 1990 Censuses' modified age, race, and sex files, 1,341,395 Indians lived in the areas serviced by the IHS. It is estimated that in the year 2000 the total population in the IHS service areas will be 1,526,000. The largest of the IHS service areas is in Oklahoma, with a total of just over 300,000 in 1998.

Throughout the Oklahoma IHS Area in 1995, there were forty-one Public Health Service/Indian Health Service hospitals and health centers (Oklahoma City Area Indian Health Service 1995). Of these, four hospitals and twelve health centers were PHS/IHS facilities, and three hospitals and twenty-two health centers were tribal facilities. Tribal facilities in the Oklahoma City IHS Area included those of the Creek Nation, Choctaw Nation, and Chickasaw Nation as well as those of the Cherokee Nation. Other tribal centers included those of the Okmulgee, eastern Shawnee, Kickapoo, Black Hawk, and the Potowatami Citizen band. Specifically, the Cherokee Nation (tribal) facilities included the Delaware District Health Center in Jay, Oklahoma; Salina Health Center; Nowata Health Center; Sallisaw Health Center; and the D. K. Martin Health Center in Stilwell.

PHS/IHS facilities serving the northeast section of Oklahoma included those of the Tahlequah and Claremore Service Units. The Tahlequah Service Unit covered a service area of some 3,400 square miles and included McIntosh, Muskogee, Sequoyah, Adair, and Cherokee Counties. Within this service area, 82.1 percent of the population was Cherokee and 8.5 percent Creek. The remaining 9.4 percent were non-indigenous people.

Facilities in the Tahlequah Service Area included: the W. W. Hastings Hospital in Tahlequah; Eufaula Health Center; Sallisaw Health Center; and D. K. Martin Health Center in Stilwell. In 1990 the Indian population (38,566) represented 22.5 percent of the total population (171,155) in the service area. During fiscal year 1994, 82 percent of the total user population (47,182) at these facilities was Cherokee (including Cherokee-Shawnee, Cherokee-Delaware, and the United Keetoway Band Cherokee). Almost 225,000 outpatient visits to these facilities were recorded in fiscal year 1994. There were 3,214 inpatient admissions.

The Claremore Service Unit was comprised of PHS/IHS facilities serving northeast Oklahoma. This service area covered just over 7,600 square miles and included the following counties: Okfuskee, Okmulgee, Creek, Tulsa, Wagoner, Rogers, Mayes, Delaware, Ottawa, Craig, Nowata, and Washington. Facilities included the: Claremore Indian Hospital (Rogers County); Creek Nation Hospital at Okemah (Okfuskee

County); Delaware District Health Center in Jay; Miami Health Center (Ottawa County); Nowata Health Center; Okemah Health Center (Okfuskee); Salina Health Center (Mayes); Sapulpa Health Center (Creek County); and Indian Health Care Resource Center in Tulsa.

In 1990, the total population within the Claremore Service Unit Area was 879,509. The largest population (503,341) resided in Tulsa County and the Tulsa metropolitan area. Of the total population in the area, only 75,618, or 8.6 percent, were Indian. The residents of the Cherokee Nation of Oklahoma comprised about 63 percent of this total. The only other group of any significant size was the Creek Nation, whose members comprised about 19 percent of the Indian population. In fiscal year 1994, the health facilities of the Claremore Service Unit registered 291,747 outpatient visits. And there were 2,402 inpatient admissions to the hospitals in Claremore and Okemah. Cherokees also comprised 63 percent of the total service population during fiscal year 1994.

CHEROKEE NATION FACILITIES

The Cherokee Nation health facilities in 1995 included the: Delaware District Health Center in Jay; Salina Health Center; Nowata Health Center; Sallisaw Health Center; and D. K. Martin Health center in Stilwell. During fiscal year 1994, the Cherokee Nation facilities received a total of 127,471 ambulatory visits. The visits ranged from over 31,000 at the Sallisaw Health Center to about 17,700 at the Nowata Health Center.

It is obvious that the PHS/IHS and Tribal health care facilities represent an important source of health and medical care for large number of Native Americans generally and for members of the Cherokee Nation in particular. From time to time, however, challenges are issued and questions are raised pertaining to who qualifies for the services: just who is a Native American? In the next section of this chapter this issue is addressed.

A PROPOSED CHANGE IN CRITERIA
FOR ELIGIBILITY

One relatively recent attempt to change the criteria for eligibility for services provided by the IHS was introduced in 1986. A notification appeared in the Federal Register published on June 10, 1986 (PHS 1986). The

Public Health Service placed a notice of action in the form of a proposed rulemaking (42 CFR Part 36) pertaining to changes to the regulations governing who may receive health services from the Indian Health Service.

Authority for the change in the proposed rule purportedly derived from a Supreme Court interpretation of the Snyder Act in a landmark case entitled *Morton v. Ruiz*, 425 U.S. 199 (1974). The Court noted, "The Snyder Act does not provide eligibility requirement or the details of any program" (415 U.S. at 208). It went on to assert that federal agencies administering Snyder Act programs had the power do define eligibility requirements and limit program benefits in accordance with rational standards.

At the time of the publication of the proposed change in eligibility for IHS health services, regulations included that: a person must be of "Indian descent" and "belong to the Indian community served" by the local IHS health facility and program. No particular degree of Indian ancestry (blood quantum) was required, and the term "Indian community" had not been defined. Thus, in the minds of the Public Health Service, the regulations had been construed liberally to include anyone who could reasonably be regarded as an Indian, regardless of degree of Indian ancestry or tribal affiliation.

At the same time, in order to be eligible for contract health services, those services purchased from non-IHS hospitals and medical providers, an individual had to meet additional requirements. The person had to be eligible for direct care under the regulations of the IHS and, in addition, reside within a designated contract health services delivery area *and* be either a member of or have close social and economic ties with the tribe located on the reservations. These requirements were more restrictive than those for direct care because contract services funds were very limited.

The established eligibility criteria had been the subject of discussion for many years within the Indian community and the Indian Health Service organization. On June 6, 1983, a notice in the Federal Register (48 FR 25273) asked for comments on a number of options for eligibility criteria. A total of 242 responses were received: 28 from tribal governments, 4 from tribal organizations, 15 from other Indian organizations, 4 from other organizations, and 191 from individuals. It was reported that the comments from individuals generally supported retention of the current eligibility requirements. The comments from tribal groups generally supported use of a blood quantum requirement for IHS eligibility, and the majority of tribes responding stated that if a blood quantum criterion were to be adopted, it should be one-quarter.

The PHS took the position that the differing requirements for direct and contracted services caused problems when patients at IHS facilities had to be referred to non-IHS facilities for care. Therefore, the PHS proposed "tightening up eligibility requirements based upon degree of Indian ancestry and residence within a defined geographic service areas" (PHS 1986). To the PHS, placing limitations on IHS and non-IHS services eligibility would enable it to provide more services with the limited IHS resources available. It would also enable the PHS to allocate resources among beneficiary groups based upon clearly defined local service populations. Finally, substituting more precise eligibility requirements applicable to both direct and contract health services would enhance coordination of patient care in IHS and non-IHS facilities.

Based upon this rationale, the PHS first proposed the "Indian and Alaska Native ancestry" be defined as meaning "descent from a member of an Indian or Alaska Native tribe that has been federally recognized by treaty or otherwise" (PHS 1986). This would establish a line of descent for purpose of eligibility, but not all persons with this ancestry would be eligible for IHS services. It was also proposed that within the above definition, persons of Indian or Alaska Native ancestry must:

> Be a member of, or eligible for membership in, a Federally-recognized Indian tribe;
> Be of one-quarter ($\frac{1}{4}$) or more Indian or Alaska Native ancestry; and
> Reside within a designated health service delivery area.

However, if a person was not a member of or eligible for membership in a federally recognized Indian tribe, then another criterion could be applied. In order to be eligible for IHS services the person had to be of one-half ($\frac{1}{2}$) or more Indian or Alaska Native ancestry and reside within a designated health service delivery area. The exception to tribal membership was proposed in order to include those who did not qualify for membership in any one tribe, for reasons such as multiple tribal heritage, but who did have a high degree of Indian or Alaska Native ancestry.

The PHS argued that those blood quantum requirements, as well as tribal membership had historically been used by Congress, federal agencies, and the courts to determine who is an "Indian" for purposed of federal benefits, claims, awards, and federal jurisdiction. Admittedly, however, there was no uniform federal standard. It was noted that "many tribes (had) recommended that we adopt this requirement" (PHS 1986).

And, "furthermore, a one-quarter (1/4) degree requirement was believed consistent with the membership requirements of many tribes." Of some 213 tribal constitutions examined by the PHS, 116 required 1/4 or more, 18 required 1/2 or more, 22 required 1/6 or more, and 7 required 1/16 or more blood quantum for membership. Fifty tribal constitutions had no blood quantum requirements as such but generally required descendency from a member listed on an original tribal roll. In addition, one-quarter (1/4) or more Alaska Native blood was generally required for enrollment in Alaska Native corporations. Thus, it would seem that the PHS was on solid historical, legal, and cultural ground in proposing some blood quantum to be used in defining Indians and Alaska Natives.

In the early 1980s, other changes in eligibility focused on the health service delivery areas. The PHS proposed geographic residency requirements to reflect the IHS obligation to Indians living "on or near" reservations and in traditional Indian areas such as Oklahoma and Alaska. It also proposed defining a new governing designation of health service delivery areas for both direct and contractual health services. The IHS would designate specific geographic areas surrounding federal Indian reservations as health service delivery areas. However, it was also the intention of the PHS to begin a reassessment of service area boundaries. For example, some of the service areas were composed of counties including reservation lands and others that bordered on the reservation. The resulting geographic configurations made a functional service area impossible. The PHS proposed to consult with the Indian tribes that would be affected by redrawing the boundaries.

The PHS also recognized that in some situations it would be inappropriate to use federal Indian reservations as the basis for defining health service delivery areas. This would be the case, for example, where there were no reservations, or they were very small and scattered, and/or the Indian population was widely dispersed. In these instances, the IHS would be authorized to designate entire states, counties, or census divisions as health service delivery areas. This would reflect provisions in current regulations that designated the states of Alaska, Oklahoma, and Nevada, as well as certain clusters of counties in Minnesota, Wisconsin, and Michigan as contract health service delivery areas. The proposal also allowed any Indian tribe located within a health service delivery area to request a change in area boundaries. The changes in definition of health services delivery areas, including input by Indian tribes and recourse for changes and exceptions proposed by PHS seemed reasonable to Indian communities.

However, by "tightening up" the eligibility requirements, some people who previously might have been eligible for free care under the rules would be placed in the "fee-for-service" category. Some people were regarded as "non-beneficiaries" under the proposed revised eligibility requirements. Nevertheless, those who lived within the health service delivery area could receive services from IHS or tribal facilities on a fee-for-service basis provided that provision of such services did not interfere with or restrict the provision of services to eligible Indians or Alaska natives.

REACTION

Indian tribes were offered the opportunity to comment on 42 CFR Part 36 before its acceptance and implementation. Because many of them already used blood quantum as a criterion in their own determination of tribal membership, on the surface the proposed revised regulations may have appeared fairly innocuous. To many, it seemed to be simply formalizing at the federal level what many Indian tribes already practiced at the tribal level.

In addition, several assistance programs already in place for some fifty years used blood quantum as a criterion for eligibility. Typically, when a person's Indian blood quantum is less than a quarter, that is, the last "full blood" was at least two generations removed from the individual, then that person might not be considered Indian for purposes of that program. Nonetheless, the blood quantum criterion had been found narrow in scope. The Bureau of Indian Affairs and the Indian Health Service had discontinued using it in the early 1980s with respect to personnel issues in the administration of their own programs.

There are at least several responses to the suggestion of using blood quantum as a measure of Indian race/ethnicity. First, there is no evidence that blood quantum has any particular sociological validity. There are no indications that individuals of lower blood quantum behave differently than those of higher blood quantum. The association of an individual with a Native American culture is determined by the specific experiences the individual has as a member of that culture. Second, regardless of its surface validity, there is a legal precedent that answers the question of whether blood quantum is an appropriate criterion for tribal membership. Third, no such requirement is utilized in determining any other racial/ethnic minority status.

GENERAL ASSESSMENT OF PROPOSED IDENTIFICATION CHANGES

Before discussing basic issues regarding the proposed changes in identification of Indians and, hence, eligibility for health care, it may be useful to point out the health status of the Indian population at the time of the proposal. The health status of the Indian population when measured by mortality ratios was considerably worse than that of the general population. For example, in 1993, 37 percent of Indian deaths occurred before the age of 45 years, compared to only 12 percent among the general population. In a number of mortality categories, the ratio of Native Americans to the U.S. population was high. The ratio was 3.1 for accidental deaths, 4.4 for deaths from liver disease (reflecting high rates of alcoholism), 5.3 for tuberculosis, 3.3 for diabetes mellitus, 1.4 for pneumonia/influenza, 2.2 for septicemia, and 1.7 for suicide (NCHS 1993).

The IHS was not serving a substantial proportion of Indians at the time the revisions in the law were proposed. This meant that rules would be put in place which had the potential to restrict the number of Indians eligible to receive services when, in fact, a large proportion already were not receiving them for one reason or another.

IMPLICATIONS

There were two important legal/moral implications in the way the IHS was proposing to define the Indian race and use that definition in the administration of its programs. First, among all population groups in the United States, Native Americans would be the only group singled out for determination of eligibility for federal benefits on the basis of race/ethnicity determined through an arbitrary blood quantum. Regardless of whether the Indians felt compelled to accept or reject this criterion of eligibility, its racial basis was both obvious and onerous (Office of Technology Assessment 1986).

Second, the imposition of federally determined criteria for race and, hence, eligibility would have taken away from the tribes the right to make their own determinations as to who belongs to their tribe and who does not. This would have been contrary to the extant Federal policy granting self-government and self-determination to the Indians. Such an intrusion did not seem justifiable in view of the fact that, historically, Indian tribes had been rather strict in their designation of tribal membership qualifications.

The most critical issue to the tribes was the question of who or what should be the appropriate authority to determine Indian status. Indians had long contended that it was a tribal right to identify who is and who is not a member of a tribe. The Supreme Court had affirmed this principle in 1978 when it asserted that it was not only a tribal right but also a responsibility (Santa Clara 1978).

Further support, if it were needed, derived from an analysis by the Office of Technology Assessment, which concluded that up to that time the federal-Indian relationship had been based on political rather than racial factors. The OTA suggested that the use of blood quanta as a basis for eligibility for health care benefits might be in violation of the U.S. Constitution (OTA 1986).

An important, though perhaps ancillary, issue of concern was related to Indian health benefits and the possible "spillover" effect of disenfranchisement. Since health services constitute a vital benefit and critical service on many reservations, the loss of benefits for those who did not have the required blood quanta might serve to push them from the reservation and, as a result, preclude their participation in Indian cultural, political, and social affairs. That is, whether intended or not, the loss of health benefits to those not qualified under the new eligibility criteria may contribute to their ultimate decision to leave or remain on a reservation. Those individuals who identified themselves as Indians and participated actively in Indian life but did not fit the federal criteria for health care benefits would likely find themselves at an economic and medical care disadvantage if they chose to stay on the reservation. They would have to obtain services on a fee-for-service basis from IHS or tribal facilities and, importantly, could be refused care should the IHS or tribal health personnel and facilities not have the time and/or space to care for them.

The definition of Indian ancestry in the proposed regulations was narrowed to include those individuals who were currently members or eligible for membership in a federally recognized tribe. Moreover, if an Indian's ancestry was traced through a tribe not federally recognized, the eligibility standard would be that the individual had to be of one-half ($1/2$) or more Indian or Alaska Native ancestry and reside within a designated health serve delivery area. These criteria were established for those persons who did not qualify for membership in any one tribe for reasons such as multiple tribal heritage, but who had a high degree of Indian or Alaska Native ancestry (Federal Register 1986).

Non-Indians who marry Indians would not have been eligible for free health services, regardless of their dependency status, with the exception of prenatal care for mothers through post-partum (about six weeks after delivery). Also, if the mother were not married, Indian paternity would have to be proven. This condition of eligibility was actually a continuation of that which had been in place since 1983.

One very serious effect of the new restriction would have been the fractionation of the family unit insofar as health services are concerned. For example, the mother (wife) who was classified as non-Indian would have had to seek health services independently, while her husband and children could have continued to utilize IHS facilities. Under some circumstances, children might even have been defined as non-Indian, even though both parents were classified as Indian.

Another important implication of the change concerned the potential economic hardship and the attendant consequences for the use of health services and reduced health status among those who would be denied benefits due to financial reasons. In addition, the selective loss of clients/patients would have had a significant impact on the service units at the local level. Service units have to be justified on the basis of the size of the service population. Below a certain number, a unit falls into danger of being closed.

Finally, the most direct negative effect of the proposed regulation would have been the actual loss of benefits for those who did not meet the new eligibility criteria. Two groups would be ineligible. First, those who were receiving benefits from the IHS would no longer be able to do so unless they could pay for the services. A second group of ineligibles would be those who were not receiving benefits from the IHS for one reason or another but primarily because they did not live in areas served by the IHS.

Importantly, data on blood quantum levels for all Indians are not available and there are substantial variations among tribes. There are, for example, tribes in the Southwest whose members are nearly full blood, with near 100 percent. And there are those with much less than 25 percent full blood living in some urban areas. In addition, there is an increasing trend among Indians to marry non-Indians at a rate estimated to be higher than 50 percent (OTA 1986). The rate of marriage between Indians and non-Indians increased about 20 percent from 1970 to 1980 (Office of Technology Assessment 1986). Therefore, in view of the changing patterns in blood quanta, the proposed regulations would have created an impossible situation for long-term planning of programs because the size of the service population, among other thing, would have been fluctuating and difficult to identify.

The notice of the proposed rule making issued by the IHS worked against Native American communities in two serious ways. First, it violated the premise of a special relationship between tribal governments and the U.S. government by usurping Congress' plenary powers with respect to Native American affairs. Second, the notice of proposed rule making was drafted prior to any epidemiological/demographic studies of the potential effects of the rules on the morbidity and mortality of Native Americans.

With regard to the latter issue, an empirical analysis of the likely effects of the proposed changes was included in an independently conducted research project (Bashshur et al. 1987). The research focused on some potential effects of the pending regulation on the Indian residents affiliated with the Clinton Indian Hospital in Oklahoma. This analysis revealed that the effects would be greatest on younger people and the children of mixed marriages, as compared to their counterparts. For those whose ancestry crossed the arbitrary one-quarter Indian blood quantum of a federally recognized tribe, the result would be an abrupt loss of benefits, with no ready substitutes, as well as the fractionation of the family whose members were no longer equally qualified for IHS benefits.

Long-term impact would include the closing of service units due to a reduction in the service population, which in turn would render the qualified residents in those areas isolated from needed health services. One conclusion of the research was that the proposed change in the regulation would "set in motion a process of ultimate termination, albeit long-term and subject to change, of providing organized health care to Indians" (Bashshur et al. 1987).

FEDERAL RESPONSE TO PROPOSED CHANGES

The proposed change in eligibility requirements met with vigorous opposition from members and supporters of Indian tribes and Alaska Native villages. For instance, the National Congress of American Indians and more than 150 tribes opposed the regulations. Some 11,000 submissions by individuals, groups, Indian and no-Indian organization, state, local, and tribal governments, and the Congress were submitted to the Department of Health and Human Services during the comment period. In addition, some 10,000 pages of transcripts taken at more than 120 public meetings held at selected locations throughout the country were obtained.

The final rule was published in the Federal Register (September 16, 1987). At that time changes were made in the rules as originally proposed. Importantly, the proposed eligibility requirement that a person must be one quarter ($1/4$) or more Indian or Alaska Native ancestry was deleted. This change was based on the comments that expressed concern that inclusion of a specific blood quantum requirement would interfere with a tribe's sovereignty by eliminating some tribal members from eligibility based upon racial identity rather than on the political relationship that exists between tribes and the federal government. Other expressed concerns were that the blood quantum requirement would: violate Indian treaty or statutory rights; shift the federal government's financial burden and responsibility to others; foster "termination"; amount to racial discrimination between Indians; divide Indian families and present tremendous difficulties involved in proving degree of Indian descent.

In light of this latter problem, the definition of Indian ancestry that specified descent from a member of a federally recognized tribe was also deleted. This was deemed necessary since it was proposed as a means of calculating Indian blood quantum. Since the blood quantum criteria had been dropped and the tribal membership requirement remained, the definition was no longer needed. Another section of the rule was revised to delete language pertaining to eligibility for tribal membership. It was determined that a majority of the respondents felt that, while opposed to the blood quantum criteria, tribal membership should be a sufficient criterion.

Thus, the federal government, based upon the response from a large number and variety of respondents, made important and well-reasoned changes, deletions, and revisions in 42 CFR Part 36. The root cause of the changes was the overwhelming opposition to using blood quantum to determine Indian identity and, hence, eligibility for Indian Health Service programs. However, additional concerns were raised among Indian groups and their supporters pertaining to other provisions in the final rule as published.

DELAY IN IMPLEMENTATION OF THE FINAL RULE

Responding to pleas that the new IHS eligibility guidelines might unfairly end medical care for many Indians, the U.S. Senate voted September 29, 1987, to impose a six-month delay on the effective date of the federal rule redefining who is eligible for IHS-funded health care services. Senator Daniel Inouye, Chairman of the Senate Select Committee on Indian Affairs, sponsored the amendment at the request of Senator Alan Cranston of California. Inouye argued that the delay was necessary in order to allow "the committees of the congress and the Indian people to seek a clarification . . . of the eligibility status of (certain) groups of Indian patients now under the care of the Indian Health Service that the final rule fails to address."

Senator Cranston asserted that the new rule would have a "devastating impact" on Indians residing in California. House Congressman Henry Waxman (California) echoed the criticism and added that the new regulations would "terminate the eligibility of roughly 50,000 rural California Indians from basic health care services." The House concurred with the Senate measure and adopted an amendment to the 1988 Interior Appropriations Bill (H.R. 2712), which pushed back the effective date of the new IHS eligibility rule to September 16, 1988.

Senate bill 2382 (U.S. Congress 1988a) was introduced as "a bill to delay the implementation of a certain rule affecting the provision of health services by the Indian Health Service." As mentioned earlier, the rule (42 CFR Part 36) was published in the Federal Register on September 16, 1987. Montana Senator John Melcher introduced the bill on May 9, 1988. On June 21, the Select Committee on Indian Affairs of the U.S. Senate held a public hearing on S. 2382 (U.S. Congress 1988b). The bill was designed to prevent IHS from implementing the regulation that would change the criteria under which Indians are eligible to receive health care from the Indian Health Service.

Senate bill 2382 stated that rule 42 CFR Part 36 should "not take effect before the day that is three years after the date of enactment of this Act, and no action may be taken before such day to implement or administer such rule or to prescribe any other rule or regulation that has a similar effect." The bill also stipulated that during the three-year moratorium on the rule, the "Indian Health Service shall provide services pursuant to the criteria for eligibility for Indian Health Services in effect prior to September 16, 1987." Further, the "Secretary of Health and Human Services, acting through the Indian Health Service, shall conduct a study to determine the impact that the final rule, or any other proposed rules which would change eligibility criteria for Indian health Services."

It was determined that such a study should be conducted with the full participation of and consultation with American Indian and Alaskan Native tribal governments, and representatives of urban Indian health care programs. The study was to include a number of items. Indian Health Service statistics pertaining to the number of Indians currently eligible would be collected. The number of Indians who would be eligible for such services if the final rule were implemented was to be estimated. The financial impact of a rule on the contract health care budget and on the clinical service budget of the IHS would be determined. There would be consideration of the health status, cultural, social, and economic impact on Indians if the proposed rule were to be implemented. Also, there would be findings pertaining to alternative sources of health care for Indians should the rule be implemented. And finally, the study would consider programmatic changes that the IHS would be required to make if the eligibility requirements for such services were modified.

Prior to submitting to the Congress the report on the study conducted under this section of the bill, the Secretary of Health and Human Services was to provide Indian tribes, Alaska Native villages, and urban Indian health care programs an opportunity to comment on the report. Subsequently, comments by these Indian groups were to be incorporated into the report.

THE INDIAN PERSPECTIVE

In addition to the study, a series of hearings were held by the Select Committee on Indian Affairs chaired by Daniel K. Inouye of Hawaii. The documentation of oral and written testimony by and on behalf of Indians against the proposed change in eligibility extends to thousands of pages in the records of Congress. Therefore, only a brief summary of the Indian response is provided here.

To many Indian people, the final proposed IHS eligibility regulations were evidence of a new "termination era," one that was administratively but not legislatively sanctioned. It was the belief of some that the new regulations would discriminate among Indians in a way that would effectively terminate members of the class of Indians. The new IHS eligibility regulations would discriminate between the class of Indians and members of all other ethnic communities by defining part of the class of Indians out of existence based on one criterion—blood quantum—a discrimination that members of any other ethnic group would never tolerate. Logan (1988) stated that Indian tribes and communities, like other minority groups, comprise indigenous minorities, which have come to include large numbers of mixed-breed and mixed-blood people (Logan 1988).

To others, the proposed change in IHS regulations represented yet another example of the "failed federal responsibility" for the health care of Indian people. Of particular concern was the belief that the new regulations would fractionate some Indian families because some family members would be eligible for care and others would not be. Examples of the special problems in this area were family counseling and immunization for children. Without counseling for the entire family, an individual's treatment may not be effective. In a family with Indian and non-Indian children, providing immunization for only the Indian children and not the non-Indian children would not produce or result in effective preventive health care. A related consideration was the increased cost of provision of care to be borne by the families. Also believed to be at particular risk under the proposed eligibility requirements were members of non-federally recognized tribes and those Indians living in areas that would not be designated as service delivery areas.

INDIAN HEALTH CARE IMPROVEMENT ACT OF 1992

The debate over eligibility for Indian Health Services programs continued and culminated in the definitions of "Indians" or "Indian" in the Indian Health Care Improvement Act of 1992. Under terms of the Act:

> *Indian*, unless otherwise designated, means any person who is a member of an Indian tribe, as defined in sub-section (d) hereof, except that, for the purpose of [sections 102, 103 and 201(c)] sections 102 and 103, such terms shall mean any individual who (1) irrespective of whether he or she lives on or near a reservation, is a member of a tribe, band, or other organized group of Indians, including those tribes, bands, or groups terminated since 1940 and those recognized now or in the future by the State in which they reside, or who is a descendant, in the first or second degree, of any such member, irrespective of whether he or she lives on or near a reservation, or (2) is an Eskimo and Aleut or Alaska Native, or (3) is considered by the Secretary of the Interior to be an Indian for any purpose, or (4) is determined to be an Indian under regulations promulgated by the Secretary.
>
> *Indian tribe* means any Indian tribe, band, nation, or other organized group or community, including any Alaska Native village or group or regional or village corporation as defined in or established pursuant to the Alaska Native Claims Settlement Act,

which is recognized as eligible for the special programs and services provided by the United States to Indians because of their status as Indians.

Urban Indian means any individual who resides in an urban center, as defined in subsection (g) hereof, and who meets one or more of the four criteria in subsection (1) through (4) of this section. Urban center was defined, as "any community which has a sufficient urban Indian population with unmet health needs to warrant assistance under title V, as determined by the Secretary.

Despite this definition, the Department of Health and Human Services stated that it does not believe that the use of a specific blood quantum cannot be precluded as a criterion for receipt of federal health benefits (Federal Register 1987). It has yet to acknowledge or recognize that determinations such as these are to be made by the U.S. Congress by virtue of the laws and court decisions, as discussed in the first section of this chapter. Since the executive branch of the federal government has yet to recognize this fact, Native American orgnaizations must be constantly vigilant and cognizant of all changes proposed by this branch of government. They must organize to oppose such changes and develop policy analysis skills and representatives sufficient to ensure that any proposed revisions are made by the appropriate body and subject to ratification by the appropriate groups within the Indian communities.

CHAPTER THREE

Communal Self-Help Concepts

The theme of this chapter is the improvement of health conditions through the assumption of collective responsibility and self-reliance. This chapter has two purposes. The first is to present a brief introduction to and conceptual analysis of self-help. The second is to assess the value of self-help as a communal strategy and rationale for health improvement by Native American organizations.

THE CONCEPT OF SELF-HELP

The concept of self-help is evident throughout history, among people throughout the world. An early writer who analyzed human and other animal societies concluded that mutual aid (a synonym for self-help) and cooperation, rather than mutual struggle and predation, enabled societies to survive and develop (Kropotkin 1939). He observed that those species in which individual struggle had been reduced to its narrowest limit and the practice of mutual aid had attained the greatest development were invariably the most numerous, the most prosperous, and the most open to further progress. Thus he concluded that in the progress of man, mutual support—not mutual struggle—had the leading part.

Before proceeding further, it is important to distinguish between the concepts of self-help and self-care, since they are occasionally used interchangeably. The two concepts refer to two different kinds of activities. Zapka and Estabrook (1975) offered a formal definition of self-care as it pertains to health. They defined it as care performed by consumers of activities traditionally carried out by providers. Continuing, the authors explained that self-care has been enhanced by the growth of "group self-help," although they did not offer a formal definition of the latter concept. Levin et al. (1976) offered a similar interpretation of self-care, later elaborated upon by Fleming (1984), "as an intentional behavior that a lay person takes on his or her behalf, or on behalf of family, friend, or community, to promote health or to treat illness." These authors clarified the concept further by raising the basic question of whether self-care is a substitute or stimulus for formal medical services. They concluded that it is a substitute.

Self-care encompasses two necessary conditions. First, it consists of individual rather than group behavior. And second, it has a clinical focus that may be therapeutic, palliative, or preventive in nature. Self-care is not a new phenomenon by any standard. Throughout history people in many parts of the world have depended upon self-care extensively to deal with a variety of health problems. This continues to be especially true of people in developing countries who have depended and continue to depend on self-care to deal with the variety of health problems that confront them on a daily basis. Similarly, though not to such an extent, people in highly industrialized societies also resort to self-care frequently (Levin et al. 1976). In some instances self-care is used as a substitute for formal medical care; however, in the majority of cases people use self-care as a precursor to seeking formal medical care. In the latter instance, self-care represents an early stage in the illness behavior process that begins with recognition of ill health and proceeds through various stages of care that may or may not involve formal medical care (Fabrega 1973).

In developed societies, it has been suggested, self-care is on the increase based at least in part on a rejection of the "medicalization" of society and the accompanying dominance of formal medical authority. Huag and Lavin (1983) suggest that "There is little doubt that renewed reliance on self treatment, both preventive and palliative, has emerged concurrently with challenge to physician authority, and is a logical extension of the public's observation that at least some medical duties can be delegated to non-physicians." They summarize the historical trends in self-care in developed societies by saying: "Whereas, in earlier times, do-it-yourself medicine and home remedies were a necessity in the absence of health care practitioners, today they are more often a choice that rejects the necessity of turning to physicians for healing." However, there is also evidence suggesting that, in some segments of society, self-care represents the continued traditions of folk medicine, persisting in spite of the availability of formal medical care.

In the literature, the definition of self-help typically focuses on group activities aimed at helping members of the group achieve certain goals. It has been referred to as "the effort of people to come together in groups in order to resolve mutual individual needs" (Withorn 1986). Katz and Bender (1976) offer what seems to be the clearest definition of self-help: "voluntary group structures for mutual aid in the accomplishment of a specific purpose." Further, they suggest that the self-help groups are formed by "peers who come together for mutual assistance in satisfying a common need, overcoming a common handicap or life-disrupting problem, and bringing about desired change."

Later, Riessman and Carroll (1995) emphasized that "self-help mutual aid groups are made up of individuals who have the same problem or need, and whose members help each other in dealing with the problem." They clarified further that "empowerment is a critical aspect of self help . . ." and that "the self-help ethos is really one thread in the new populism that is beginning to affect the political scene." Riessman and Carroll also state that "self-help movements reflect the new bottom-up politics." Katz (1993) suggests that self-help groups that engage in sociopolitical actions to effect policy changes for the benefit of members and nonmembers alike are important not only for the ends achieved but also because the social action becomes a unifying force for the group. These issues will be taken up later in the chapter.

Katz (1993) suggests that the idea and expression of self-help always reflect and respond to broad social developments and changes. Social class, educational levels, attitudes toward minorities, and the degrees of democratization, decentralization, and local autonomy as they exist in different societies strongly affect both acceptance of self-help groups and the particular forms that self-help assumes. In addition, although the social and group dynamics of self-help development may be broadly based, self-help groups originate, in part at least, from the psychological basis of human behavior.

The driving forces of this behavior have been identified as needs. One of the most influential theories of human motivation is that of Abraham Maslow (1970). He attempts to integrate psychoanalytical insights about conscious and subconscious processes with other biological and social factors. Maslow's well-known analysis places human needs or drives to behavior in a hierarchy or pyramid of five major categories.

The most fundamental need or drive is comprised of the physiological needs such as hunger, thirst, and the need for sleep. These become the most basic needs in times of extreme external stress or deprivation. Next comes the need for security or personal safety, both physical and psychological. This group of needs results in behavior that removes or reduces personal fear and anxiety as well as physical threats. This behavior can be accomplished at the level of the individual as well as the group by providing reliable social arrangements such as law and order for protection of the individual.

Individual behavior cannot be separated from any of the categories of needs posited by Maslow, and his third need category has been identified as most directly pertinent to the self-help field—the need for affiliation, affection, and social acceptance. These needs drive individuals toward the group for support and recognition. Coupled with the previously identified physiological needs for safety or security, as well as the need for esteem and self-actualization discussed below, the basic motivation for attaching oneself or developing a self-help group is realized.

Maslow's fourth category is the need for esteem, which includes self-esteem as well as the esteem or regard of others. Both have been identified as motivations for affiliating with self-help groups. His fifth and final category is the need for self-actualization, that is, the need for self-fulfillment, the fulfillment of one's potential. In an ordered world, this need and behavior related to it emerges only when the first four categories have been achieved. However, it is important to realize that from time to time the order of importance of the needs and, therefore, behavior categories may be temporarily rearranged. At times behavior related to the need for self-actualization may temporarily become dominant. Early participants in the civil rights movement, for example, subjugated their safety and security for self-fulfillment of the individual and the group.

ATTRIBUTES OF SELF-HELP

Two related attributes of self-help are its collective structure and the assumption of responsibility for mutual helping. Self-help, as such, constitutes a group or a communal response to problems faced by a collectivity of individuals, and it uses group reinforcement to assert collective responsibility. Moreover, to the extent that professionals become involved in self-help activity, they do so to assist not only clients and their families, but also and perhaps more importantly, to develop support networks and to sponsor programs. Therefore, self-help is different from "professional helping' because only the former requires private effort and communal responsibility (Lieberman 1979).

The assumption by the community (as a collectivity of individuals) of a certain level of responsibility for a common problem is a critical component of self-help. When this activity occurs, the benefits to be accrued by the group are not debatable, regardless of political or social ideology. That is, when group members work together for the purpose of providing or satisfying an important need in the community, everybody benefits. Communal collective efforts produce benefits for everyone in the community, those who are engaged directly in the effort and those who are not. However, the aim of self-help in health and other matters is to encourage all affected individuals to participate in the collective process in order to maximize the benefits for the community as a whole. In some instances, the original focus is multiplied as more individuals and problems are brought into the process.

The women's health movement is one such example. While the modern, late-twentieth-century movement has gained considerable notoriety, its roots may be traced to the Ladies' Physiological Society of the nineteenth century (Morantz 1977). The Society originated in Boston in the 1840s and soon spread to other cities. Its initial focus was women's health interests including pregnancy, childbirth, and child rearing. The Ladies' Physiological Society campaigned and educated women to promote better nutrition and self-care during pregnancy, including the wearing of less restrictive clothing, "natural" childbirth in the home, and the rearing of infants and toddlers according to folk wisdom, which diverged from the prevailing medical and religious dictates. The Society not only advised women on these aspects of day-to-day behavior, but it also dispensed a philosophy that parallels that of contemporary feminism. It acknowledged the positive influence of women in society and the family, which led to a re-examination of the relationship between the sexes and a rejection of the authoritarian concept of marriage in favor of marriage based on mutual love, common interests, and affection (Morantz 1977). Currently, one of the most notable examples of organized multipurpose self-help movements is the women's health movement. It is concerned with educating women about their physical and mental health, redressing the exploitation of women by the medical care system, establishing referral sources, as well as providing resources to protect women against all forms of abuse at home and at work (Boston Women's Health Collective 1973).

The current consumerism movement can be cited as another contemporary and corollary movement that also has achieved some level of success in representing consumer interests. Many organizations were created to combat high prices, monopolistic price-fixing, shoddy workmanship, "planned obsolescence," and the marketing of hazardous products. In contrast to earlier consumer movements, these groups could provide scientific and technical analysis of widely publicized products. This has been accomplished through media exposure and public education, which helped bring about a higher level of consumer consciousness than had previously existed.

The present day consumer movement has had some of its most notable and successful activities and effects in the field of health care and health products. These successes stem in part from the publication of health data, evaluation of the needs of disadvantaged groups, and mediation or instigation of various types of action (Haug and Lavin 1983; Katz 1993). Many of the health-related self-help groups have adopted or developed a "consumerist stance." Health oriented groups raise the consumer consciousness of their members in several ways. First, they evaluate institutions and individual professionals according to the care and knowledge of the problem they offer. Second, they evaluate the cost and effectiveness of products on the market including drugs, appliances, and so forth. Third, they often deal with legislative policy issues, joining with consumer activists and other citizen groups to support or oppose particular legislation or policy proposals.

On the basis of the preceding discussion, we can make an operational distinction between the two closely neighboring concepts of self-care and self-help. Self-care largely refers to what individual people do in the process of illness behavior when they recognize a deviation from the normal state of health as determined by a reading of the biological system or when acknowledged by members of their family or other reference group. Self-care refers to what people do for themselves when they do not feel the need or the appropriateness of consulting a professional provider. Further, self-care is confined largely to responses to clinically oriented kinds of interventions, whereas self-help incorporates a broad range of communal activities. Self-help generally consists of an organized activity undertaken by the members of a group (or the formation of a group) for the purpose of resolving or ameliorating problems faced by the entirety. To be sure, there is at least one common element between the two concepts, namely the assumption of responsibility by the individual or group for their own care and/or for promoting conditions that affect the individual (group) well being or health. Our interest here, of course, concerns self-help activities pertaining to the improvement of health.

Another concept can be incorporated, with some justification, into the discussion of self-help to explain the case illustration considered here. That concept is community development, which typically involves a broader range of activities than self-help. In that sense and under certain conditions, communal self-help may be viewed as part of community development, especially when both efforts are directed toward a common goal or toward resolution of the same problem. Yet community development cannot be part of self-help under certain conditions because the former is broader in scope than the latter. The underlying reason for the preference of the Cherokee Nation of Oklahoma to use the term communal self-help rather than community development is largely historical. The term *community development* derives from programs developed in the 1960s as part of the largely failed "war on poverty." It may be argued that community development continues to be an active concept. However, the Cherokee Nation of Oklahoma and other Native American organizations believe that reviving and relying on images of the war on poverty are unlikely to help their efforts to revitalize their communities through self-help.

More importantly, the concepts underlying community development are not totally applicable to the special status of American Indians and Alaska Natives. For instance, it has been suggested that the most significant theory derived from community development was "maximum feasible participation" (Rubin 1969). This may appeal to the disenfranchised poor and minorities, but it is an anathema to the Native Americans. It is far less than what they believe is their right, namely, self-determination. When used in this context, the concept of maximum feasible participation embodies at least two troubling aspects for Native Americans.

First, Native Americans believe that their rights should not be considered in the same manner as the needs of the poor. In other words, meeting or complying with these inherent rights should not be dependent upon the federal government's "largesse." They believe that Indian participation in the planning, design, and implementation of programs aimed to serve them should not be limited to the principles embodied in the concept of maximum *feasible* participation. This is especially true considering the vagueness with which this term has been defined. It is very troublesome to Indians to be accorded what they feel are their rights only to the extent that it is "feasible" to any extent.

Second, and especially germane to the topic of this chapter, the notion of community development is too broad. It tends to involve several dimensions or multiple foci that preclude or are beyond the scope of a single, focused self-help activity. Hence, the Cherokee Nation of Oklahoma has emphasized the concept of self-help whenever it could. What it and the other Native American organizations stand to gain, without risking any losses in control or legal rights, is individual responsibility for promoting conditions conducive to good health in their communities.

THE IDEOLOGY OF SELF-HELP AND HEALTH

One of the most interesting aspects of self-help is its ideological orientation, representing a group function aimed at problem solving. Self-help has a factual basis in terms of specific sets of behaviors undertaken by a group. At the same time, it has a normative content in terms of shared responsibility and collective effort. In this section, the ideological orientation of self-help will be discussed, primarily the polar dimensions related to the question of private, or individual, responsibility versus that of the public sector for health conditions.

In the United States, "good health" was considered "most important" by one third of the people in a national survey, second only to a "loving relationship" (Gabel et al. 1989). The concept of health as a private or individual responsibility and enterprise is widely held in Western culture. The majority of the population in the United States, for example, probably would agree with (but, perhaps not put into practice) the notion that individuals should assume a primary responsibility for their own health. This would include such things as adopting healthy life styles and using suitable health services when it is appropriate to do so. Evidence to support the former can be marshaled from, however temporary, the proliferation of health clubs, growth of the food supplement, vitamin, and personal health equipment industries, and the expansion of health promotion/disease prevention programs in the workplace.

It may also be reasonable to assume that only when individuals demonstrate an incapacity to deal with a health problem or when there is a need for collective response to problems such as cigarette smoking or industrial pollution should public agencies intervene. The logical conclusion of this viewpoint embraces the notion that most illness is the consequence of individual vulnerability or failure. Problems of ill health are viewed, at least in part, as consequences of individual/community failure to behave in appropriate ways to prevent illness and disability, or a failure to promote health and well being.

Friedson (1970, 1976) addressed "common sense individualism" and suggested the possibility of two flawed assumptions underlying the concept. The first is denial of the existence of a stable, structured environment that "constrains, limits and channels" individual behavior, thereby reducing the capacity for individual control over behavior. The second possibly flawed assumption is that the "individual's characteristics are formed at some point in time into a stable and fixed bundle of knowledge, motives and values," so that behavior (the response to Maslow' needs) will always be guided by this bundle—regardless of environmental conditions. In reality an individual has very little control over some illness-producing situations in the environment. And an individual's behavior is governed not only by conditions of the external environment but by an incomplete, imperfect, complex, and changing set of knowledge, beliefs, and motives.

From the other side of the equation, the argument has been made that public agencies should assume responsibility for creating healthy environments, promoting health life styles, and assuring health care to all individuals (Knowles 1977). From this perspective, health and health care constitute basic rights of citizenship, and therefore the responsibility for providing health care in order to assure health moves from the individual to the government. Problems of ill health are attributed to the failure of the system (or public agencies) to assure a healthy or at least benign environment, provide incentives for health behavior, and directly provide services to individuals who cannot get them privately. Taken to its logical conclusion in this scenario, individual responsibility for health is abrogated to the government and a federally mandated medical care system. Individual health and illness behavior becomes the responsibility of the government and public agencies. Of course, one potential problem in this system is that it assumes that the government knows what is best for the individual's health and health care, and further, that the medical community can and will provide only that medical care which is appropriate and necessary.

In response to a perceived growth of this phenomenon, a number of critics became alarmed at the "medicalization of society" (Illich 1976). Concern was expressed over the abrogation of individual control and responsibility and the encroachment of the federal-medical complex into medical as well as non-medical aspects of life (Fox 1977; McKeown 1979). Illich (1976), a staunch proponent of that position, suggested that illness and health had been expropriated through the government by the medical profession, which was depriving individuals of their right to experience the reality and individuality of their own existence. The overwhelming rejection of a 1993 federal attempt to take over the health care system in the United States indicates either the strength of opposition to government intervention of this magnitude or a seriously flawed federal health care proposal (Wollstein 1993; National Center for Policy Analysis 1993).

Meanwhile, other health reform advocates have criticized the modern U.S. health care system for exploiting illness for profit (Ehrenreich and Ehrenreich 1970; Navarro 1976), for having limited and dubious impact on health (Carlson 1975; Knowles 1977), and for discriminating against certain segments of society (Corea 1977; Sidel and Sidel 1984).

In the United States, the decade from 1990 to 2000 has witnessed a rapid rise and proliferation of managed care in the form of health maintenance organizations and preferred provider organizations. Increasingly, these forms of care are also coming under considerable criticism for the control such organizations exercise over the enrolled individual's choice of physicians and hospitals. Physicians employed by these organizations also complain about restrictions placed on their freedom to explain medical care options to patients as well as about constraints placed on prescribing treatment.

Yet it is clear that health and health-related problems form the basis for development of the large percentage of self-help groups, indicating that resources beyond the medical care/government sector are needed. Health-related self-help groups are often created when a number of people identify a common health need that is not being met by existing organizations and that, they feel, can be addressed by joining together. A New Jersey study of self-help groups, for example, found that in 1988 the largest number of groups was formed to help individuals with mental-health problems (Leventhal et al. 1990). The second largest number of self-help groups formed was for people with Acquired Immunodeficiency Syndrome and their family members, and the third largest was for relatives of people discharged from mental hospitals.

Within the context of self-help, the debate over the specific role of the private sector or group of individuals vis-a-vis that of the public sector (or its surrogates) in dealing with health issues raises a number of fundamental policy questions. The primary one is how to reconcile individual and public and/or government responsibility for health (Riessman and Gartner 1984). The tension or balance and resulting strain between individual (or private sector) responsibility for health does not fully account for the rise of self-help groups. Sometimes self-help groups are organized to resolve problems perceived to be beyond the reach of existing public programs or the services available through the professional medical care sector—and certainly, when an individual perceives that the problem cannot be met alone. Katz (1993) suggests that the creation of new self-help groups is obviously related to social conditions. As new social problems emerge that affect particular groups or classes of people, problems which apparently are not being taken care of in other ways, formation of new self-help organizations is to be expected. However, the development of self-help groups is not dependent upon "new" problems, those not yet considered or addressed by the private or public sectors. Self-help groups are also responsive to long-standing problems and issues that, for one reason or another, are either ignored or beyond the presumed scope of the private or public sectors.

Robinson and Henry (1977) suggest that the development of self-help groups in society derives from impetus provided by: (1) the failure of existing services to meet public expectations; (2) the wide recognition of the value and benefits of mutual self-help; and (3) the dissemination of information about self-help through the cosmopolite (mass media) or through personal means. Accordingly, the decline of traditional supportive social institutions and the failure of professionals in handling an increasing number of everyday problems lead to a discrepancy between needs and resources. Thus, the creation of self-help groups is the "natural" response to serve a recognized need.

The role of "anti-professionalism," or the rejection of resources, services, and programs designed to meet the needs of individuals, as an impetus for the development of self-help groups is a matter of debate. Some disagree with the notion that self-help group formation is related to anti-professionalism (Lieberman 1979). They point out the significant role played by professionals in the development of self-help groups and the fact that members of self-help groups frequently utilize professional services more than non-members. Further, it has been suggested that individuals might serve as "effective advocates for professionals" given the appropriate conditions and situations. Of immediate interest is the possibility that a greater emphasis on self-help (the assumption of communal responsibility for health improvement) might result in an increased demand for professional health services as a necessary complement to a comprehensive health program.

Professionals are concerned that certain characteristics of self-help groups may, in fact, be hazardous to the individuals and community involved. This is by no means a new opinion, but the volume of critical commentary on this issue has increased considerably with the rise in professional and self-help interaction (Katz 1993). Professionals worry that self-help groups will create new problems or even intensify those problems that may be too difficult for laypeople to handle unaided. The source of this concern is the potential spread of misinformation and the adoption of simplistic solutions to complex problems.

Other concerns of professionals include evidence that some group leaders regard themselves as professionals in their own right, fully capable of dealing with complex and technical issues. As such, these group leaders may discourage group members from consulting qualified professionals when necessary. Some professionals fear that groups may "shop around" to compare the performance of institutions, personnel, and facilities, thereby impugning the status of professionals. Clearly, these latter concerns reflect the potential challenge that self-help groups pose to the often-monopolistic position and self-perception of professionals and established institutions.

THE RELATIONSHIP

Given the concerns and the often contentious issues raised by professionals and self-help groups about their relationship, it is to be expected that a number of ideas have been proposed to ameliorate or resolve them. In a relatively early observation on self-help groups and mental health professionals, it was observed that they were "made for each other," that they share a common purpose and do essentially the same job (Gartner and Riessman 1980). The guiding principle derived from this observation is that the dissonance between the two can be resolved by educating each group about the other and increasing interactions between them (Katz 1991; 1993). This formulation's assertion that professionals and self-help groups do essentially the same things for clients or members and therefore are interchangeable fails, however, in light of the peer group influence and the sense of community generated by and within self-help groups. Rarely, if ever, is a professional a "peer" in the sense of having personal experience with a problem or being personally identified as a member of the group or community. The idea that both types of services are necessary for a given problem may also be called into question. In some situations self-help groups alone can be very effective and even sufficient. In other situations technical or professional input is essential and may be a prerequisite for developing and maintaining an effective and efficient self-help program. Regardless, self-help groups organized and conducted by laypeople have a different character and function than those created and led by professionals. The powerful element of peer support, the effects of individual role models within the group, and the interactions occasioned by the giving and receiving of help have been identified as distinguishing characteristics of the "non-professional" self-help groups. Included among other distinguishing factors are the socialization of the group experience, the proximity of group members to "everyday life," concern with the present, and development of spontaneous personal relationships. There is a growing realization that professional help, no matter how competent, sensitive, and well-meaning cannot supply these benefits (Katz 1993).

Professionals must be cognizant of the differences and value inherent in self-help groups organized, managed, and run by laypeople. They (professionals) must understand what laypeople know and what they can accomplish for themselves and their community. Much of this understanding must come from a respectful attitude and from interaction with self-help groups. Given the fear and prejudice among many professionals toward self-help groups and, in turn, suspicions among laypeople toward professionals and the fear of co-optation, there is much ground to be covered before a mutually satisfactory working relationship will be achieved. Nevertheless, it seems certain that we will see more contact between professionals and self-help groups, greater cooperation and research toward problem solution, and along the way, an enhanced respect for the special knowledge and experience that each side possesses.

SELF-HELP, EMPOWERMENT AND POPULISM

To be sure, the concepts of empowerment and new populism have been two of the more significant characteristics of the self-help movement, especially within the past several decades (Riessman 1985; Katz 1993). Empowerment refers to a sense of control and individual autonomy and control over personal affairs. It relates to characteristics of personality, cognition, and motivation and is expressed in an individual's feeling of self-worth and of being able to make a difference (Stewart 1990). Empowerment, in fact, has become a very popular shorthand way to describe the purposes of many social movements. It is clear that empowerment of members of self-help groups, sought consciously or not, does occur. This is true especially within the more successful and lasting groups.

Examples of populism in the United States can be found back in the mid-nineteenth century. We have already discussed, for example, the Ladies' Physiological Society, which originated in Boston in the 1840s. Self-help principles were also embodied in other nineteenth-century political and social organizations that came to be known as the American populist movement. Prior to the Civil War, populist organizations were created among farmers and rural populations and among small merchants in the towns, especially in the South and Midwest.

A detailed examination of the populist movement is beyond the scope of this chapter. Suffice to say that the overall objective of populist groups/organizations was to build resistance to political domination by the federal government in Washington, D.C. and to oppose the economic power of big businesses, banks, and other financial institutions. In the agrarian sector, farmers established cooperatives for the production and distribution of food, for example, building warehouses to store crops until prices became favorable. They loaned money at rates below those charged by banks, purchased equipment, and marketed their goods and products. And, they took political action to accomplish their goals. Interestingly, in some southern states the alliances even embraced black farmers, who had been ostracized from political life there since Reconstruction.

These initially economic-based populist organizations parallel what takes place in self-help groups formed around a single condition or issue (Katz 1993). One observer (Goodwyn 1976) writes that "perhaps the most significant institution of the Populists—one that they came to learn from their own organizing experience in democratic movement building—is that once people agree to work together for an agreed-upon goal, the experience of working toward that objective has the effect of raising their sights by transforming their understanding." Indeed, the Populist movement became politically significant in national politics and peaked in influence in 1896 when William Jennings Bryan, a Democrat who sympathized with the Populist agenda, won his Party's presidential nomination. Sacrificing its independent identity after Bryan was defeated, the Populist Party faded steadily from the political scene.

The populist spirit in American did not disappear, however, and the social action methods employed by today's self-help groups, though diverse, are similar to today's populist, grass roots groups. They stress education and put pressure on politicians through lobbying, public demonstrations, delegations, mass meetings, and media coverage. New populism is reflected in what is perceived to be a pro-community, anti-big business/anti-government attitude.

It may be argued that empowerment runs the risk of becoming dogmatic, though its effects may be perceived as concrete and undeniable. Indeed, it can be argued that individuals tend to prefer to solve problems on their own. This idea runs counter to the notion that government should be the source of corrective measures related to social problems identified by groups of individuals or suffered by segments of society. And among those government institutions and political parties whose livelihood depends upon "doing for" groups of individuals in need, the proliferation of self-help groups poses a threat similar to that perceived by professionals. In fact, it has been observed that one positive outcome of the self-help movement's questioning of the role of government has been the development of a neo-populist movement. In this movement, "government is defined as the agency of the community providing useful and necessary tools, neither the enemy nor the solution" (Katz and Levin 1976).

A number of approaches have been used (some by the government and professional groups) to engender a feeling of control over conditions that affect health. As such, empowerment and neo-populism have become significant contributors to the promotion of confidence on the part of individuals, groups, and communities. This confidence reflects the realization that it is possible for the average person to understand personal health status and related problems, and to know or learn how to marshal and use resources effectively toward improvement. Through self-help activities this confidence can be instilled and developed.

THE CHEROKEE SITUATION

The history of Native Americans and the special relationships between Indians and the federal government complicate the concept of self-help and community development among the Cherokee Nation of Oklahoma, as well as other Native Americans. Two issues, namely federal responsibility and dependency, must be addressed if the concept of self-help among Indians is to be fully understood.

FEDERAL RESPONSIBILITY

One of the most important duties of the U.S. government is the responsibility for natural and financial resources that the Secretary of the Interior holds in trust for American Indian tribes (Lujan 1991). For almost 150 years, law and tradition have assigned the Secretary of the Interior the responsibility of carrying out the federal government's trust obligations to the American Indians. As mentioned earlier, over the past 200 years the Indian policy of the federal government has vacillated between the extremes of paternalism and termination. Paternalism materialized as the maintenance of Indians on reservations; termination conversely sought to abolish tribal governments and reservations, allotting land to individuals and forcing Indians into mainstream American society. Each of these extremes have been imposed on Indians, and each proved disastrous for Indians.

Over the past several decades, since 1970, a new Indian self-determination policy has been in effect. Purportedly, at the core of the self-determination policy is a deep and genuine respect for American Indians and the important role that tribes have played in forging a strong, multicultural nation. This policy encourages tribes to maintain and perpetuate their rich cultures and heritage. At the same time, it permits tribes and individual Indians to join the political, economic, and social mainstream of modern society as they see fit. An additional basic principle of self-determination is a government-to-government relationship. The federal government deals with tribal governments much the same as it deals with state and local governments.

This policy also reaffirms the federal government's commitment to continue providing services directly to tribes under the treaties, laws, and court decisions that govern Indian affairs. And, importantly, the policy also encourages tribes to develop the capability, through funds from the federal government, to take charge and operate social programs in such areas as education, safety, and health. Under this policy, pilot programs were initiated that enabled qualified tribes to assume more control over the full package of federally funded programs serving their members. Rather than providing prescribed sets of federal programs to tribes, the federal government offered each tribal government the opportunity to shape the package and to see that the services were delivered to their members. In effect, the tribal governments were taking over the full range of functions that had been performed for a century or more by the Bureau of Indians Affairs agency and area offices.

Whether the philosophy has been one of paternalism, termination, or self-determination, the fact remains that the ultimate responsibility for Indian affairs lies with the federal government. Though the term "self-determination" makes it sound as though Indians have the right to administer their own affairs, develop projects, and distribute resources as they see fit within their society, the reality is that they are not permitted to succeed or fail on their own accord, learning as they move toward true independence, true self-determination, and self-governance. Some tribes are sophisticated, with a competence at least comparable to that of the most efficiently run city or county government. Other tribes, however, have yet to develop the expertise to fully deliver the broad array of services now provided by the Bureau of Indian Affairs and other federal agencies.

Regardless of the level of perceived sophistication, the ultimate arbiter and overseer of "self-determination" among Indian tribes is the federal government. Not all who speak of self-government mean the same thing by the term (Ambler 1991). Self-government and self-determination mean that decisions are made not necessarily by the people who are wisest, ablest, or closest to Washington, but rather by the people who are most directly affected by the decisions. Thus, the context and framework for the development of self-help and communal development among Indians is not equal to that among other segments of the population. Fundamentally, we cannot assume that we have the answers and that Indian tribes do not. The rights and responsibilities of self-determination and self-government belong to the tribal governments. They have the capacity and certainly should have the right to make their own decisions and, at times, their own mistakes.

POSITIVE DEPENDENCY

It is clear, therefore, that along with the notion of ultimate federal responsibility, the issues of dependency must be addressed when considering self-help among the Indians. At first, the issues of self-help and dependency seem contradictory. Dependency is a sensitive subject, considered an automatic negative by many in an American culture that seems to stress individualism and independence (Gurian 1977). But dependency should be and often is considered a positive in traditional cultures.

Dependency operates between individuals, between individuals and groups, between groups and groups. It crosses time and space lines. In dependency, the individual or group seeks support, identity, security, or permission from outside entities. In the case of the American Indians, this type of dependency has been imposed by and resides in the federal government. The direction of dependency interaction is reciprocal: the dependent seeks, expecting that which he depends upon to respond. This type of relationship necessarily creates a bond between the two entities. The respective weltanschauungs, or worldviews, of the groups involved determine the nature of this bond, which may be constructive (positive) or destructive (negative).

From the Euro-American perspective, the negative bias toward dependency can be traced to a post-Renaissance worldview that emphasizes the psychological and political rights of the individual against the obligations of the individual to larger units such as family, group, sect, or state (Gurian 1977). Certainly American colonists practiced mutual aid, because in small communities neighborliness was necessary for crop planting and harvesting, for house building, and for protection against "hostile native Americans and other settlers" (Katz 1993). However, the fertility and availability of land and the absence of centralized, oppressive state controls made mutual aid less necessary in America than in Europe, and the American ethos of "making it" through individual effort soon developed. The progress of science and technology, too, created the means for functioning as independent units and as a culture that supports this type of behavior. As defined largely in Euro-American terms, dependency is a necessity in infancy, which the "healthy" personality sheds as a part of the maturation process (Snyder 1963; Gurian 1977).

Again, it is crucial to realize that the Euro-American worldview has set the tone and shaped expectations pertaining to Indian behavior. Meanwhile, given a different environment and mindset, Native American people have expressed independence within a larger framework of lifelong dependence. That is, they have developed (and develop in) a culture where ancestors, elders, or guardian spirits judge them. Their lives require cooperation at every point, so that on an everyday basis, the Native American life is based on the need to interrelate for survival. Myths reflect this understanding, while the perception of the cosmos help them to depend on dimensions beyond those measured by the senses. Indians were part of a cooperating universe and therefore psychologically "threatened" by situations in which support could not be found. This "positive dependency" is basic to myths, stories and customs of hundreds of Native American tribes and is as fulfilling as the independence of the Euro-American without supervising structures.

As discussed in an earlier chapter, the rise of the Cherokee Nation in the mid-1700s was an instance of independent face-to-face communities joining voluntarily (Gearing 1961). Within the villages, the Cherokee consciously distinguished between two categories of tasks and villagers organized themselves as personnel differently when they attended the tasks in each category. Red tasks involved such things as war, negotiation with foreign powers, and ball games. These were coordinated by a command through a hierarchy of war ranks under the village war chief. White tasks, on the other hand, included ceremonials, councils, and agriculture. These were coordinated by voluntary consensus that was created through the influence of the elder men in their respective clans, all under the leadership of the village priest-chief who was both the symbol of village harmony and the major cause of that harmony.

Thus, the apparent contradiction between the American Indian development of self-help and its dependency upon the federal government can be resolved. Such an arrangement, combining traditional integrity with traditional dependence, makes sense to most Indian people.

The rise of self-help among the Cherokee Nation of Oklahoma, therefore, came about as a natural extension of the historical traditions of positive dependency, and the routine process of communal decision-making and cooperation (Fogelson and Kutsche 1961). That is, when the community was faced with a common problem, in this case the need for safe water and effective waste disposal systems, it was reasoned that the solution had to stem from members of the community. The selection of this case study to illustrate Cherokee self-help for health improvement is predicated on the well-founded assumption that these utilities are critical for good health, perhaps even more so than the opening of a new clinic or organization of a disease-specific support group.

CHAPTER FOUR

The Cherokee Self-Help Experience

This first section of this chapter briefly describes some of the cultural traditions within the Cherokee Nation of Oklahoma, providing the context for the development of the self-help movement. This is followed by a description of the process of communal self-help within the Nation as it pertains to the development of a public health infrastructure—specifically, here, water and sewer systems. The selection of safe drinking water and effective waste disposal systems among the Cherokee as a case study in self-help for the improvement of health is predicated on the assumption that these utilities are critical to the collective good health of a community. As such, the specific case illustration of water and sewer is used primarily as a vehicle to illustrate the process by which the project was developed, rather than the mechanics or the technical requirements for installing the system. Again, the focus is on the process of self-help rather than the project per se. The final section of the chapter assesses this specific instance of the Cherokee experience of self-help within the context of the general principles of self-help, discussed in the previous chapter, as well as within the traditions of the Cherokee culture.

The potential usefulness of this discussion depends upon the extent to which it demonstrates to American Indian and Alaska Native organizations the merits and policy implications of the methods employed in establishing and nurturing communal responsibility for health improvement. The fundamental lesson to be derived from this illustration is that the success of a communal self-help project to address a collective problem can build competence and confidence. From such a beginning, communities can embark on more complex self-help projects focusing on health improvement. The ultimate objective here is to promote the concepts of self-reliance and local control, as well as the basic tenets of self-help as a viable approach for improving health conditions in local Native communities.

PROPOSED FRAMEWORK FOR ASSESSMENT

The starting point in the development of a conceptual self-help framework for health improvement was to identify the roles to be played by members of the Cherokee Nation of Oklahoma as well as by non-members. The focus was on pinpointing activities appropriate for members of the local community as well as the roles that would be functional for "outsiders," including public agencies, professionals, and/or technicians.

Personal health status can be viewed as constituting a continuum from perfect health at one end to seriously ill health (and ultimately death) at the other. Individual responsibility should be greatest under conditions of good health, while the individual has significant control. In other words, an individual has the responsibility to engage in healthy behaviors, or those behaviors that help maintain the current level of good health. This would include, for example, exercising, maintaining a proper diet, and avoiding behavior that places good health at risk, such as smoking or excessive consumption of alcohol. In the face of obvious symptoms of ill health, the individual should act sensibly and responsibly. That is, the individual should respond to "readings" of health status provided by physiological, psychological, and social subsystems that indicate a serious negative change in health status has occurred. In the presence of such symptoms or readings, the individual should take appropriate personal action and should seek competent help when indicated. The individual must want to get well. The individual (and the community) has certain rights and responsibilities when it comes to health behavior (preventing ill health) and illness behavior (remedying ill health when it occurs).

Viewed from this perspective, behaviors related to the onset of illness, and the steps taken to correct or eliminate the illness, are comprised of a series of stages. The stages include: (1) recognition that a significant negative deviation in health status has occurred; (2) identification of the problem; (3) evaluation of the potential seriousness (and cost) of the illness; (4) consideration of alternative strategies for rectifying the unfavorable situation; (5) selection of an initial treatment plan; (6) evaluation of the impact of the plan; and, (6) if the outcome of stages 1-5 is unsuccessful, a recycling through the previous stages in the process.

Ultimately, when faced with a serious illness that is not alleviated by personal actions and local resources, the individual must seek assistance and medical attention from professional sources. In this scenario, the individual has a responsibility to follow the directives of medical professionals. This is not to imply, however, that the individual assumes an entirely passive role during this stage of the process. Indeed, much to the dismay of some medical professionals, the individual is encouraged and indeed may have the responsibility to be an active partner in the professional medical care process. The individual should seek to understand not only the nature of the illness but also the nature (potential benefits and side effects) of proposed treatments. Under conditions of poor health, therefore, while the individual retains some personal responsibility, the amount of personal control over the process, though limited, is still extant and presumed essential to a successful outcome.

Individual experience informs the self-help communal experience in that self-help works best when individuals have input and maintain ultimate control. Moreover, a clear-cut division of labor or abrogation of responsibility is not assumed; the individual can and should play a significant role in all stages of health and illness behavior. Of course, this assumption does not pertain to the unconscious individual or, by extension, to the community that has suffered a disaster that renders it completely beyond effective and meaningful participation/input into the resolution of the problem. The public, or institutional, sector can play a positive role in promoting healthful life styles, providing a safe environment, and protecting individuals and groups from unscrupulous health or medical practices and harmful products.

Therefore, certain elements of responsibility lie with the individual/group/community and others with professionals and the government under almost all conditions of health and threats to health. The roles and the amount of responsibility vary with each circumstance. This realization is useful for considering the amount of emphasis or for determining primary responsibility appropriate to a particular set of circumstances, rather than apriori considering individual/community versus public/professional sector roles as exclusive jurisdictions. The challenge for policymakers is to determine what can be done to promote individual/community responsibility without withholding public responsibility and accountability where it is appropriate and necessary. The challenge for the individual/community is to determine the point at which it is necessary and appropriate to engage the public/professional sectors and the level of input from these sources. At the same time, the individual/community must deal with the issue of locus of control. Again, these situations with regard to Native American communities are complicated by the special position of dependency of these groups on the federal government and, in turn, the federal government's responsibilities to them.

CHEROKEE BELIEF SYSTEMS

The effective use of various resources, including medical care and facilities related to improvement of the public health, requires clarity and understanding of those values and beliefs pertinent to the community's aspirations. One of the most important aspects of the self-help movement within the Cherokee Nation of Oklahoma was the recall and clarification of as well as recourse to the traditions of Cherokee society, including health and health care. Recognition of these beliefs proved to be critical to the development and the eventual acceptance of the self-help program. When concern arose within the community that some individuals had lost touch with the beliefs underlying development within the Cherokee culture, the leadership took the time to remind the people of them. A detailed narrative of the Cherokee traditional societal and "medico-magical" beliefs and practices is beyond the scope of this chapter; however, a brief summary will inform the reader of aspects of Indian culture that are relevant to any implementation of self help and that need to be addressed.

The early acculturation experience of the Cherokee has been recognized as atypical compared to the general model of acculturation for most North American Indian groups. Of course, this is primarily due to their geographic location relative to, and almost continuous contact with, the first European settlers. One of the aspects of Cherokee culture most resistant to change has been the medico-magical practice (Fogelson 1961). The invention of the Sequoyah syllabary in 1821 was as a powerful instrument of cultural retention. Conjurors, formerly dependent upon oral transmission, transcribed sacred formulas and other lore into notebooks.

During the earliest recorded period of contact, the Cherokee medico-magical beliefs were mediated through a stratified priestly organization that was observed to be both pragmatic and flexible prior to the Removal. While many American Indian groups had definite notions of supernatural power in their ritual and vision quests, a clearly defined power concept was not so conspicuous among the Cherokee. Throughout Cherokee history, there has been a decided disinclination to set oneself above one's fellows. Cherokee ceremonialism, and in fact much of the Cherokee personality, seems oriented toward harmony with nature through knowledge and control, rather than through blind supplication.

Importantly, the highly esteemed medicine men, as well as other guardians and interpreters of traditional belief were among the Cherokee forced to emigrate to the West. Obviously, the shock of removal, separation from their homeland environment, and the experience of the "trail of tears" resulted in some loss of culture. However, it also resulted in a more compulsive adherence to those items of medico-magical belief that survived. In 1961 it was observed that "only with the intensive culture contact of the past 25 years [that is, since 1936] had Cherokee medico-magical practices begun to undergo major accommodative modifications" (Fogelson 1961). In general, the impact of Western medicine on Cherokee theory and practice was seen to involve partial assimilation, the accentuation of difference where the two theories were irreconcilable, and an overall recognition that the two systems were complementary, rather than fundamentally contradictory.

The modern Cherokee Nation of Oklahoma was developed upon a somewhat modified traditional cultural system enforced by a new life style. This necessitated development of what has been termed a "reservation culture" (Goggin 1961). Most importantly, however, to a large extent this "new" cultural development is an adaptation of the traditional belief systems carried by the Cherokee from their original homelands. These, in turn, were influenced by the early contact with Europeans.

It has been observed that any action that is taken among the Cherokee is first discussed in a leisurely, informal context by groups of people. A kind of consolidation of sentiment emerges. Then the matter is brought up in a formal context, usually by an older person with some prestige in the community, for the group's consideration. Any decision on this formal level requires some semblance of unanimous agreement.

A crucial element of the traditional Cherokee worldview involves seeing the universe as having a definite order, as a system that has balance and reciprocal obligations between its parts. The individual Cherokee is part of this system, and so membership entails certain obligations. When each Cherokee does not fulfil these obligations, the system gets out of balance and the Cherokee no longer have the "good life" (Thomas 1961). Thomas observed in 1961 that this worldview had remained stable and continued to impact upon any action taken by the Cherokee. Further, the Cherokee leaders were conscious of this philosophy and tended to weigh problems in light of this formulation. It was within this framework that the modern Cherokee Nation of Oklahoma undertook the self-help effort.

COMMUNITY DEVELOPMENT ACTIVITIES

Community development activities began in the mid- to late 1970s. They came about as a result of the desire by employees of the newly formed Cherokee Nation government for resources to be focused on those who resided in "rural, full-blood communities." In other words, the original attention was focused on those who lived within the context of the most traditional of Cherokee values. These communities contained the highest levels of unmet social and health needs, and it was assumed that these communities held the greatest potential for a successful implementation of a self-help approach because of their very adherence to traditional values—and the compatibility of self-help with these values.

The process by which the self-help-based development of a safe water and sewer system was pursued by the Cherokee Nation of Oklahoma involved five distinct steps. While self-help was conceived as a process consisting essentially of these steps, there was some latitude in terms of the relative emphasis placed on each, as well as flexibility regarding other details of implementation. The five steps are listed below.

Step 1: Conduct a survey and rank-order the importance of the needs or aspirations as identified by the community.

Step 2: Explain and discuss problem(s) underlying the identified need(s) and/or barriers to achieving the goals.

Step 3: Discuss who should be involved in the resolution of each identified problem.

Step 4: Discuss alternative solutions/strategies and achieve a consensus on the selection of a particular approach.

Step 5: Implement the intervention as agreed upon by members of the community.

These steps are not unlike those many have tried and are what most would agree to be the logical way of engaging community self-help strategies to solve common problems. What may be different about the approach of the Cherokee Nation of Oklahoma are the techniques used for completing each step.

NEEDS ASSESSMENT

The first step, in all instances, was to ask community members to describe their needs and aspirations. Subsequently, the Nation's leadership held a series of local meetings in the communities to discuss the issues, allow input from the members, and to achieve a consensus on identifying problem areas. Generally, people initially identified those problems and issues that they thought "outsiders" wanted or expected to hear. Also, in these forums, community members commonly did not make a clear distinction between problems versus needs. For example, the prevalence of gastroenteritis and other intestinal illnesses represented a community problem, whereas, clean water represented a requirement for alleviating the problem. Given this situation, therefore, it was soon realized that it was important to develop a method of community self-assessment, through which community members discussed the issues among themselves, rather than before a group of outsiders.

The community's needs were then stratified according to a determination of whether they were basic to survival or "merely" provided an enhancement to current living conditions. Care was taken to see that (a) an excessive (and disconcerting) amount of time was not spent distinguishing between needs and enhancements and that (b) where appropriate, community aspirations were distinguished from more individual interests. The role of the Cherokee Nation leadership in these activities was to facilitate the discussions at the local community level.

Additionally, the leadership exercised great care in order not to raise expectations from the needs assessment process itself, lest those expectations lead to frustration and disappointment. This approach derived from previous experience wherein similar efforts culminated in results well below unrealistic expectations. For example, certain activities that were designed to generate new revenue failed, and instead of being income-generating, became income-draining activities. The ultimate impact was demoralization of community members about the specific activity and, perhaps just as important, a loss of enthusiasm for future community development activities. Acknowledging the importance of not over-selling the needs assessment process, at the same time it is important to not "undersell" expectations, lest enthusiasm for those projects subsequently proposed wane from this direction as well.

Local communities were given full control over their own needs assessment. In all instances, the role of the Cherokee Nation staff was limited to assuring that the methodologies employed conformed to applicable standards and were consistent across projects. Local residents made all other decisions regarding the assessments. They conducted the needs assessments, with technical assistance from the staff of the Cherokee Nation of Oklahoma on an as-needed basis. In the case of the water/sewer needs assessments, one of the most commonly identified needs, assistance was provided by the Community Development staff in each community. In the case of health status surveys, local health departments provided the assistance.

PROBLEM DESCRIPTION AND EXPLANATION

One of the most commonly identified needs within the Cherokee Nation communities was that of clean water. It was quickly and widely recognized that source identification, transportation, and storage of clean water were very technical matters. Moreover, while the need was common across the communities, the individual community problems with these matters were considerable. Therefore, the second step of the self-development process, problem description and explanation, was conducted within each of the communities. Community meetings were held to discuss the needs, problems, and possible solutions in specific communities. This step recognized the individuality of each community and its needs, and avoided the common problem of "one size fits all" solutions crafted by federal agencies in response to needs and problems identified within the Cherokee Nation of Oklahoma.

In this second stage, local community leaders and community members requested assistance from the Cherokee Nation of Oklahoma in the form of technical experts and consultants to help with the process. Wherever and whenever possible, the Cherokee Nation directly provided that technical assistance. When the necessary and appropriate technical consultant or expertise was not available within the community or the Nation, Cherokee Nation staff assisted the communities in identifying and acquiring help from appropriate outside sources.

The objectives of the meetings were to reach a common understanding of the need and its related problems and to arrive at a consensus on the value of trying to address and ameliorate it. While this second stage of the self-help development process was tailored to each community, the meetings in which the problems were fully described and discussed followed a relatively standard format. The reason for doing this was to give local residents the opportunity to describe problems associated with the need as well as perceived problems in meeting the need. A full and open discussion was encouraged and, if necessary, more than one meeting was held in order to ensure that every community member would have the opportunity to participate in discussions.

Subsequent to the discussions and questions raised by community members, the appropriate technical expert or consultant, such as a sanitation engineer or construction specialist, was given the opportunity to address the issues and questions raised. These consultants, informed of the local situation, then explained, in whatever depth necessary and appropriate to the question, why the problem existed and the scale and types of difficulties that might be encountered in resolving it. Also addressed and provided were alternative solutions and their associated costs and time frames. Finally, and most importantly, the local residents were informed about how they could contribute to and participate in the resolution of the problems identified.

Following these initial discussions and presentations, local residents were encouraged to ask questions to clarify points brought up during the meeting or to raise any additional points not yet considered. Community members discussed among themselves, as well as with the consultants and technical experts, the relative merits of the various approaches that had been identified other issues perceived to be pertinent. It was considered very important that a local member of the community facilitate these discussions. In some cases the individual was a recognized leader from the community and in some instances it was not. Often, more than one individual would be involved in facilitating the discussions. Frequently, the facilitators would have a special interest in a problem or issue and/or be conversant with the problem or issue being addressed. In many cases, therefore, the individuals facilitating the discussions would turn to be someone "unexpected" from the community, that is, someone not directly or actively involved in the particular issue.

THE ISSUE OF PROBLEM "OWNERSHIP"

The mainstay of the Cherokee Nation's approach to self-help was the emphasis on problem ownership. The basic question here revolved around whose need or aspiration was being addressed. To answer this question, the working assumption was that a community "owns" a problem when: (1) its existence is recognized by or derived from sources within the community, and (2) the community develops and feels a responsibility to solve it. The common experience of many Indian communities with regard to community development has been that "outsiders" perceive a problem within the Indian community, target (define and delimit) the problem, design a solution for the community independent of significant community involvement and traditions, and, finally, implement or impose the solution. Within the process as perceived by the Cherokee Nation of Oklahoma was a firm belief that there would be little chance for effective and permanent change if community members did not directly relate to (identify with) the problem and its solution.

There are three widely accepted views as to why a community fails to "own" a problem. (1) Past experiences may have conditioned a community to look to others to assume responsibility for identifying a need/problem, developing a strategy to meet the need or resolve the problem, and marshaling outside resources to implement the strategy or solution. Thus, in this scenario, which has been enacted many times in the past, the community and its members have been excluded from meaningful participation, so that over time a negative type of dependency became inculcated into the community. (2) Within this framework, it became easier to blame others for problems than to assume direct responsibility for them, and (3) the reliance on outsiders became as expected as the exclusion of the involvement of the community and its leaders.

The Cherokee Nation of Oklahoma developed four approaches to encourage local ownership of problems. The first was to eliminate or discourage the idea of the existence of a rigid formula for success. Emphasis was placed on the process rather than the outcome. Therefore, consideration of the process became standardized in terms of basic steps, but the specific solutions were acknowledged to vary from problem to problem. In this scenario for community self-help, recognition is given to any individual within the community who brings new ideas to the table that enhance the understanding of a situation and/or the resolution of a problem.

The second approach has been to make community development and progress dependent upon the local community's work and decisions. The community and its members are expected and, in fact, required to bring input into the identification of needs, developing a priority of needs, understanding problems related to meeting needs, devising alternative strategies to resolve the problems and, finally, taking an active role in implementing the strategies. This was necessary in order to counter the negative dependency culture that had developed among large segments of many Native communities.

The third approach was to ensure that the solutions were both manageable and personal. Communities would be discouraged from direct involvement if the solution to a problem were perceived as overwhelming in terms of scope or complexity. Projects were subdivided into several linear segments or phases. This increased the understanding of each among the members of the community. And as each phase was completed, a sense of fulfillment was achieved and greater confidence was instilled in community members' ability and capacity for self-help.

The fourth approach was to see to it that owning the problem meant getting credit for its solutions as well as accepting responsibility for set-backs. This was a sensitive issue and had to be addressed carefully. Of course, it was easy to give credit where credit was due. However, when the implementation of a proposed solution was not successful, it was necessary to acknowledge this also. The manner in which this was done was to emphasize the iterative nature of the solutions to most problems. Rather than assigning blame for failure, the approach involved looking at the problem again, that is, revising the identification of the problem or the approaches and the merits of various alternative approaches. This is analogous to the situation of an individual who, having initially identified an illness based upon a given set of symptoms, sets out several courses of action to resolve the problem. When a selected course of treatment fails, often the problem has to be revisited or redefined and an alternative strategy selected. There is no blame involved in select-ing the "wrong," or what turns out to be an ineffective course of treat-ment. Rather, it is simply acknowledged that problem solutions are not "cut and dried" but often require the testing of alternative strategies before the correct or most effective one is selected.

ALTERNATIVE SOLUTION STRATEGIES AND SELECTION

The principles involved in solving the problems were basically the same as for those related to identifying ownership of the problems. The most difficult stage in the process was allowing the community to make the selection of the various problem resolution strategies suggested. It had been common for outside technical advisors and consultants, openly or unintentionally, to identify one among many acceptable alternative strategies as the "best." This would sometimes result in friction between the consultants and community or among community members them-selves. Thus, the meeting(s) in which a strategy or potential solution was decided upon offered the most opportunities for things to go wrong.

Despite the best intentions, there was a strong potential for the indi-vidual providing technical assistance to dominate the process. This was viewed as a critical stumbling block to the development of com-munity ownership of a problem. Any problem, though identified by the community, can diminish in value or urgency should the community not see its own solution applied to or as an option toward the resolution of the problem.

Because of its importance to the entire process, staff representatives of the Cherokee Nation of Oklahoma tried to co-facilitate solution and strategy selection meetings with the local residents. While it did not guarantee success, this cooperation was viewed as minimizing the potential of a solution strategy imposed from the outside and maximizing the potential for community ownership of the proposed solution. The desired outcome was a consensus (bordering on unanimity) on the strategy or solution selected to be employed, the formation of a work committee that would take the lead in planning the project, and agreement upon the time frame within which the work would be completed.

IMPLEMENTATION

The fifth and final step in the community self-help process is implementation. One of the decisions made by the Cherokee Nation early in this process was to ensure that the developmental work was conducted in the self-help mode. This led to two additional principles being adopted that would govern the activity. First, the Cherokee Nation would only work in those communities into which it was invited. And, second, any community that invited Cherokee Nation participation in the process had to be willing to invest a significant and meaningful proportion of the resources necessary to complete the project.

The majority of projects in the first decade of community self-help development were centered on water/sewer systems and housing. Implementation was accomplished in a truly communal self-help fashion, in which community members contributed time, effort, and scarce and valuable financial resources to develop and install the systems.

Though not documented with empirical data, a number of benefits have been recognized as accruing from improving the water/sewer systems of communities within the Cherokee Nation of Oklahoma. Among the more significant benefits are those related to cost of construction, community maintenance and support, and finally, confidence in and expansion of community self-help efforts.

According to informal evaluations by the Indian Health Service, water/sewer systems within communities of the Cherokee Nation of Oklahoma engaged in self-help were built for about 40 to 50 percent of the costs of similar systems built in neighboring Indian communities in northeastern Oklahoma. In other words, between 2 and 2$^1/_2$ times as many miles of equal water/sewer lines had been put in place in the self-help communities for the same amount of money spent by non-self-help communities.

Another benefit derived from the self-help experience has been the development of expertise in the construction and operation of water/sewer systems within the community. The educational experience garnered by community members in the design and construction of the water/sewer systems has paid dividends in terms of maintenance of the system. When part of the system needs repair or replacement, in many instances the necessary expertise and skills can be found within the community. This has reduced dependence on outside contractors and it has resulted in a system that has significantly less down time and, therefore, more consistent and continuous operation.

A third benefit also derives from the self-help nature of the development of the sewer/water systems in the communities. Since the communities are well aware and informed as to how much the system cost to build and maintain, and because the system is theirs, they have been more than willing to make the monthly payments for the water/sewer service. This is unlike other communities in which a system was designed and built by outsiders. In these communities suddenly a person receives both a connection fee and a monthly water bill. In the self-help communities, in contrast to others in which water/sewer systems have been installed, the bill collection rate has been very high. According to program records, the collection rate in the self-help communities has been consistently above 95 percent—a rate far exceeding the programs that did not employ self-help.

Finally, and perhaps most importantly, the successful implementation of the self-help water/sewer projects has had a significant impact on other areas of health improvement. In the self-help communities, the level of confidence regarding their ability to identify and meet other health needs seems to have been substantially increased. These communities have come forward both more frequently and more confidently with requests for assistance in addressing other local health problems. The Nation wants to ensure that the principles of self-help form the foundation of these requests and become the normative behavior in the communities. Therefore, rather than responding immediately to increasing numbers of requests, the Cherokee Nation of Oklahoma asks the communities to follow the principles and guidelines established by the self-help experience. In other words, communities need to identify their health needs, develop a priority for addressing each need, develop (with assistance where necessary) a range of alternatives, and select a specific strategy for meeting the need(s). In this way, the Nation hopes to foster further the notion of self-help within the communities and build on the successes of the initial water/sewer self-help projects.

IMPLICATIONS OF COMMUNITY SELF-HELP IN THE HEALTH SECTOR

The success achieved in addressing safe water and waste disposal problems by employing a community self-help strategy affected not only the communities involved. The Cherokee Nation as a whole was affected as well. Indeed, the Cherokee Nation seized the opportunity to acquire more control from the Indian Health Service over the provision of health services. Thus, the concept of self-help has transcended the local communities within the Nation and now functions in the larger Nation.

The Cherokee Nation of Oklahoma has eschewed assuming managerial responsibility for in-patient services (an alternative available to it). Instead, the Nation chose to manage those programs that are most sensitive to traditional cultural values and beliefs. These include health education/promotion programs; community nursing/health workers and home healthcare activities; and supplemental food programs for women, infants, and children, as well as the poor; mental health and alcohol rehabilitation programs; and selected outpatient clinical programs.

The Nation outlined a series of goals related to reduction of infectious and chronic diseases, compliance with treatment protocols for such things as diabetes and hypertension, as well as reduction of health risk behaviors such as smoking, excessive consumption of alcohol, and obesity. As in the case of other self-help developmental work, the emphasis in the health programs managed by the Nation has been to solve problems rather than just manage them. Gradually, the Nation has been assuming responsibility for such programs from the Indian Health Service. While they do operate independently from the community development activities, the overlapping, interdependent nature of each becomes increasingly evident. And importantly, the need for expansion of the principles of the self-help process becomes evident.

For example, because the Nation and the Indian Health Service had been providing services in the communities for decades, it seemed unnecessary to determine new or unaddressed needs of the communities. It was common knowledge among both the Nation and the IHS that cancer and heart attacks were the leading health problems. Nonetheless, they agreed to assist the communities in conducting a health survey. Once the community self-assessments were completed and the results assessed, it became obvious that diabetes and hypertension were the leading health problems, not cancer and heart attacks. Indeed, the prevalence of diabetes among adult males was estimated to be 40 percent. Thus, the initial step in self-help, self-assessment of needs, was instrumental in revising common knowledge and, most importantly, instrumental in laying a foundation for community (Nation) ownership of the problems. Thus, it became far more effective in the long run for the communities and their members to inform not only the Indian Health Service but the leadership of the Cherokee Nation of Oklahoma as well, that, in fact, "These are our problems."

As in the case of the water/sewer programs, with regard to diabetes the second step in the self-help approach was to bring in appropriate medical experts to address the local community members about the problem. Though it was uncommon for an extended family not to have at least one diabetic member, it was equally uncommon to find local community members with adequate levels of knowledge pertaining to the symptoms and sequelae of diabetes. An endocrinologist from the IHS was invited to community meetings at which members described their concerns and listened to descriptions of the problem and alternative interventions to address the problem. At subsequent meetings in the communities, the various strategies were discussed and initial remedial actions selected. Once more, the involvement of the IHS and the Nation were secondary to the active role of the local community.

An important distinction can be made between those communities addressing the problem of diabetes. Among those with experience in the self-help community development programs, there is a greater assumption of individual and community responsibility for the type of strategy selected and the expectation that the problem can be addressed and resolved within the confines of the local community and its traditions. Conversely, in communities in which there have not been self-help projects, members have assumed a lower level of responsibility and maintain a greater expectation that the solution to this health problem resides with health care providers.

LAYING THE FOUNDATIONS FOR FURTHER SELF-HELP

The Cherokee Nation of Oklahoma used a self-help approach for the development of community water and sewer systems to lay the foundation for individuals to become more involved with efforts to improve their health. Once the efficacy and effectiveness of the self-help approach were demonstrated in the development of this public health infrastructure, members of the respective communities that had adopted this mode of mutual cooperation and control moved on to similarly develop programs for diabetes and hypertension.

While understanding the belief system of the Cherokees provides an appropriate framework for pursuing specific improvements in conditions of health, it does not provide the instrumentality by which they can be pursued. Nonetheless, they can be limited to the generic components that should be considered in implementation. One specific example was described here, a large-scale project to provide safe running water and sewage disposal in all villages lacking this important health infrastructure. The Cherokee Nation of Oklahoma leadership utilized this project as a catalyst for change, not only for the purpose of achieving the specific and immediate objectives, but also for reinforcing traditional beliefs and establishing a common framework for addressing other problems that need to be resolved. They promoted the idea of incorporating self-help in all developmental projects to be undertaken by the community. Thus, rather than viewing the need for a safe water and sewer system as independent of other needs, the Nation tried to capitalize on the need for developing an effective strategy to meet other components of their economic, social, educational, and health needs as well. The key to success is making self-help self-sustaining.

THE IMPLICATIONS OF SELF-HELP

In some ways the development of a self-help movement among the modern Cherokee Nation of Oklahoma mirrors the experience of non-Indian groups in their efforts to gain control over their life experience and to correct problems identified as important to the collective group. But as we have seen there is a unique legislative and legal context within which this movement is being developed here. A number of Cherokee traditions were carried to Oklahoma along the Trail of Tears and, though suppressed by many years of oppressive and regressive government policies, have been rekindled and become conducive to the self-help experience and movement. And in turn, the self-help movement may be viewed as essential to the survival of the Indian culture itself.

As discussed earlier, throughout the early period of their recorded history, the Cherokee people demonstrated a communal approach to the identification and solution of shared problems. This has been observed at several levels. Indeed the rise of the first Cherokee State in the mid-1700s is considered an instance of independent face-to-face communities joining together voluntarily. The common problem faced by the Cherokee people at that time and for many years was the incursion of European settlers into Cherokee territory and their seemingly unquenchable thirst for Cherokee land, a problem that continued even after the removal (Gearing 1961).

In the face of this continued threat, the Cherokee also proved remarkably adaptable, incorporating European educational and economic systems and developing a new and vital cultural mix of tradition and progress (Waldman 1985). Coupled with this adaptability, however, has been a strong tradition of independence. For example, the Cherokee along with the Choctaw refused to acknowledge the Dawes Severalty Act of 1887—better known as the General Allotment Act—whereby Indian reservations were to be broken up and the land allotted in parcels to the heads of Indian families. The ultimate goals of this strategy were to increase the amount of land available for white settlers and to eliminate Indian communities and culture. In this instance, as in many other instances, the Cherokee turned to the American legal system for redress, only to be thwarted by congressional intervention.

In the face of repeated attempts over the past 200 years to destroy the Indian culture generally and the Cherokee culture specifically, the Cherokee and other Indian tribes somehow have persisted and emerged once again, albeit with an inevitably modified and complex cultural base. These cultures appear to be the result of a highly selective process of adoption, interaction, and invention of culture traits. The result is a live, adaptive, and highly integrated system of behavior, belief, and technique fitted to life in a specific environment and age.

In 1961 a rather pessimistic perspective on the future of the Indian "reservation culture" in America was presented in a symposium on the Cherokee and Iroquois cultures:

> Perhaps the most important phase of reservation cultures is what is happening to them today. The problems which Indians face today are the same ones all of us face—problems of community survival and progress, problems of preserving some personal integrity despite rapid culture change, problems of ego survival in the face of powerful threats to personality. Reservation cultures are making so much greater a transition in entering the modern world and in coming to share in a modern cosmopolitan culture, that the threat is indeed overwhelming. The immediate future holds little promise, for we see too little progress in community betterment, too much discontent, too poor a public health picture, too little economic betterment, growing social fragmentation, culture loss rather than replacement, and increasing production of aberrant personalities. These can be deadly threats to any community anywhere, but they are especially severe forms of threat to the reservation community.
>
> (WITTHOF 1961)

It is from this scenario that the Cherokee Nation and Indian communities across America are trying to escape. While community self-help is not the magical "silver bullet" that will resolve the larger problems and threats they face, it can be seen as a valuable weapon against the loss of Indian culture in America. The Indian communities represent important national resources in population, vigor, individualism, and philosophy, if only the people can find their place in American life without the vast losses in personality and spirit.

CHAPTER FIVE

The Negotiated Investment Strategy

This chapter describes a program adopted by the Cherokee Nation of Oklahoma, the Negotiated Investment Strategy (Strategy), which was designed to coordinate the formation of strategic plans for the development of an effective social infrastructure. Also discussed in this chapter are ways in which other tribal or small governments could adopt, in whole or modified, the strategy. In keeping with the purpose of the book, the primary focus of this chapter will be to suggest approaches for the development of effective health policy among Native American organizations and communities.

The many and sundry governmental units and agencies in the United States, ranging from villages and towns through state and federal governments, direct significant portions of their budgets to the development of social and economic infrastructures and toward alleviating perceived problems in these areas. Generally, these are problems that the private sector is unable or unwilling to address on its own. Within the health sector, the problems typically revolve around, but are not necessarily limited to, disease prevention and therapeutic medical care programs for the indigent; emergency medical services; mental health care; and programs directed toward improving the environment. Yet, regardless of the level of government being considered, it is rare that the departments within them that are responsible for these services coordinate the services or strategically plan for their development and delivery.

Often assistance from external or outside sources is provided on a categorical basis, and most frequently, the categories of services provided in this manner derive from the provider or donor's perception of the local need or its own priorities for funding projects. As discussed in the preceding chapters, this perspective often does not match the perceptions and actual problems of the local community, and the result can be a dissonance between those providing the service and those toward whom the service is directed. While in many instances such assistance is both seriously needed and appreciated by recipient groups or communities, often discord and distrust can develop within the provider-recipient relationship. Through such tensions in the relationship, not only are the potential beneficial effects of offered services not maximized, but disharmony caused by a lack of coordination and the frequent development of competition between outside and local groups can manifest in negative results.

There continues to be a significant gap between the health status of Native Americans and that of the general population. One of the reasons is the failure to coordinate and integrate those health services already available to them, as well as the failure to coordinate and develop a unified strategy for the planning of additional services. While crucial to the situation among Native American communities, the situation is not unique to them. The federal government recently recognized the problem existing within one department, the Department of Labor (Department of Labor 1995). Problems in coordination and communication between the department and the pubic sector, between the DOL and other departments, as well as between agencies within the DOL itself, resulted in an attempt to "reinvent" the process of rulemaking and implementation through a process called Negotiated Rulemaking.

What may be unique to the Native American case is that even during times of fiscal and program retrenchment and downsizing, there may be too many (albeit uncoordinated) rather than too few services being provided and made available to program beneficiaries. Moreover, even under these conditions, the Indian experience has been that service providers fail to take advantage of the potential benefits of coordinating and sharing services and resources. The providers also fail to recognize that Native Americans would benefit from operation efficiencies and the potential synergies derived from a well-designed strategy for organizing and integrating developmental programs and services. Examples of previous service duplication and restrictive regulations experienced by the Nation include three separate community-based energy savings programs serving portions or all of a local area population—each with its own program and staff. The uncoordinated multiple programs, which focused on a single problem, were in direct competition with each other and, as well as being inefficient, absorbed extraordinary and substantial administrative costs. Also, due to specific regulations pertaining to use of vehicles for transportation, potential clients of educational social service programs and programs for the elderly were unable to obtain the transportation needed to travel to service providers because the vehicles were restricted to use by clients of each specific program.

SOURCES OF THE PROBLEM

As illustrated above, the lack of coordination and integration of services is obviously not a problem limited to the health sector or to social development within Native American communities. It is common to departments and agencies responsible for providing services and resources to the communities. Nevertheless, there may be several specific factors that account for the failure of the Native American communities to realize and achieve savings and increased benefits from the coordination of services. These reasons are presented and briefly discussed here to help clarify the issues and, more importantly, to set the stage for proposing ways of redressing them. The reasons include *externality, categorization, territoriality, invested inertia,* and *dispersal.*

Externality

In most, if not all instances, for the majority of Native American communities, ideas for new programs have come traditionally from sources external or outside the community. These usually take the form of a government agency or private foundation initiative to redress an externally perceived need among the people. In the absence of self-help infrastructures among the Indian communities, in many instances, the externally perceived problems and their perceived level of priority may not match the perceptions and priorities held within the community itself. Additionally, this directed externality results in a failure of the private donors or government granting agencies to communicate and coordinate among themselves, let alone with existing local representatives and programs.

An illustration of this problem would be an outside organization providing grant or other funds to address problems associated with child abuse. Often the local units toward which the funds are directed and that would ultimately utilize the funds are not included in the planning or administration of the grant on a shared or coordinated basis. Thus, the local department of social services, which was there before the grant, will continue in place during the period of the grant, and will remain subsequent to the grant's termination, does not play an active role. This situation can lead not only to an inefficient use of resources, but can affect negatively the status of the local department and those responsible within the community.

Categorization

Categorization means that externally generated and derived assistance usually comes to the community on a categorical rather than a global basis. That is, frequently, the assistance is narrowly focused, and funding is allotted for limited use, whereas a more effective use of the funds would be to direct them to related problems not included in the categorical funding. For instance, external support for a health program is rarely linked with another program dealing with a related human service need, such as education. Thus, representatives of the agencies/donors of categorical funding for health will rarely sit down with educators to do strategic thinking and negotiate the framework and limits of the health service initiative. The result is often a fragmented and, therefore, a less effective approach to problems that are in reality interrelated and in need of comprehensive solutions.

Territoriality

The third factor, territoriality or "turf," may be a contributing factor to categorization discussed above. Territoriality or turf, which may be more prevalent than generally admitted, refers to the existence of what might best be referred to as "feudal systems" or vested interests among the government agencies and private donor organizations. In the private sector there are frequently two or more groups with similar interests, for example, child nutrition. If these groups are competing for donations, there is little likelihood that the management staff of each will cooperate or coordinate with the other. Similarly, government agencies compete for a pool of funds allocated from one budget period to another, and they jealously guard their territory or area of responsibility. Frequently, agencies within different departments have programs developed to address the same problem. Yet to cooperate and coordinate their efforts would mean a reduction in budget. In the opinion of each agency, this is to be guarded against "at all cost"—and the cost is frequently lack of communication and cooperation. In both the private and public sectors, therefore, fragmentation or categorization of planning (or maintaining the status quo) is in their best parochial interests.

It should be mentioned here that the notion of territoriality also exists at the local level in many communities. Responsibility for a problem and control or power over a given set of resources contributes to efforts to resist coordination and cooperation in addressing a multi-faceted problem. Thus, the same problems related to territoriality among external agencies and donors can be found as well within and among local agencies and departments.

Invested Inertia

A fourth factor to be considered relative to the lack of cooperation in areas of problem development and planning is resistance to change within organizations, even when that change might be beneficial to them. The more comprehensive the proposed change, the greater is the resistance it. It has long been observed that changing "organizational characteristics is inherently difficult" under any condition, and especially when the changes are sweeping (Katz and Kahn 1966).

As an illustration, Wilson (1998) has spoken recently of "consilience" as a key to unification among the domains of learning and as essential to targeting, understanding, and resolving some of the more important issues facing us today. Wilson focuses his initial discussion on the academic world. In this sector, by consilience, he means the "lumping together" of knowledge by "linking facts and fact-based theory across disciplines to create a common groundwork of explanation." To accomplish this, however, would mean that the current boundaries of the academic disciplines would have to be dissolved and a common language and set of goals established. The imagined resistance to even this largely hypothetical challenge to the invested inertia of each academic discipline is daunting.

The concept of consilience can be extended to the arena of funding and granting agencies and organizations. By linking areas of concern and strategies to redress problems, a much more effective and cost-efficient approach to resolving identified problems could be achieved. However, these organizations and departments have different authorities upon which they base their programs and, hence, different strategies for approaching problems within their purview. Unfortunately, they have different strategies for resisting change and adopting the concept of consilience, too. This, in turn, is often cited as a principal reason why certain organizations (departments) cannot coordinate their strategic thinking with other organizations (departments).

Dispersal

A fifth factor that inhibits coordination of programs is the functionally and geographically dispersed nature of the concerned and/or appropriate parties. This is especially the case on reservations and in rural areas and increases the difficulty of involving all that should be involved. It is not a simple or straightforward process for funding and/or granting agencies to determine apriori all the potential beneficiaries from a given program. Adding to this problem is the substantial geographic distance between potential recipients and, thus, their relative isolation from one another. In the past it has not been uncommon for some tribal programs to discover and be surprised by the fact that other tribal programs have been established in the same area for a period of time. Often it is not only the organizers and agencies but the recipients of services as well who do not have a full understanding of the distribution of need and the programs already in place.

PROBLEM IMPLICATIONS

Having identified a number of problems pertaining to the lack of coordination within and among programs regardless of the source, the next issue concerns the potential implications of the problems described above.

There are at least four notable implications, including *inefficient use of resources, diminution of program impact, lack of synergy,* and *disenchantment.*

Inefficient Use of Resources

An inefficient use of resources is brought about by the lack of a coordinated strategy, resulting in unnecessary duplication of programs and services and therefore the waste of material, money, and effort. In certain circumstance, the lack of a coordinated strategy results in dis-economies of scale or even lost opportunities. The Cherokee Nation felt that the potential dis-economies of scale were probably a greater source of concern than duplication. Indeed, the Nation was not overly concerned about having too many services because it felt that this type of problem could be remedied and handled relatively easily.

The greater focus of concern on the dis-economies of scale derived from the experience that, for the most part, programs were not funded to provide an adequate amount of service. The Cherokee Nation administrators felt, therefore, that the failure to properly combine and provide services resulted in unacceptably high average total and per capita costs. Their view reflected the fact that as long as each program provided only a limited quantity of service, each would be operating at points on the average cost curve where appropriate efficiencies would not be experienced.

Diminution of Program Impact

A second negative outcome of uncoordinated program development and service provision is the serious diminution of impact or effect. When not funded adequately, programs simply cannot work well and do not achieve the desired impact on the target population or problem. This is not a matter of inefficiency; rather, it is primarily an issue of failure to achieve the critical mass of services necessary to be effective. For instance, a substance abuse program funded at one-half the necessary amount achieves less than one-half of the desired effects of a fully funded program. To be effective the approach to substance abuse requires a full spectrum of services ranging from institutional care for physical detoxification, institution-based care for social detoxification, continuous ambulatory care and case management, as well as community based educational services. In addition, general education and employment are also critical factors in addressing substance abuse programs in the community.

Most of the past efforts in this area have been designed to address only one or two dimensions of the problem and, therefore, have resulted in predictably inferior outcomes. A physical detoxification program, for example, without an anti-substance abuse education program may result in a high rate of recidivism. And recidivism itself may lead to frustration for the client and even greater substance abuse. This is only one example of why non-comprehensive, uncoordinated efforts are not efficient. The narrowly focused programs may be efficient internally, but the impact is less than in coordinated ones; there may be negative consequences inherent within them; and they have a higher per capita cost.

Lack of Synergy

Narrowly focused or one-dimensional programs are less than the sum of their parts. When services are not coordinated, the synergism that normally results from coordination and integration of efforts is lost. The problem is then "what did not happen" as a result of an uncoordinated and less than comprehensive efforts. While it might appear as a truism, it should be stated that a coordinated, integrated program strategy that provides a comprehensive range of services tends to produce results greater than the sum of the individual parts when the parts are implemented singly. For instance, an early childhood education program integrated with a health promotion/disease prevention program(s) will result in broader and more positive outcomes than when one or more of the programs are implemented independently.

Disenchantment

A fourth negative outcome of the lack of a coordinated strategy is disenchantment. This result is rarely acknowledged but is known to many policymakers and community leaders and members. Disenchantment has to do with the manner in which community leaders and members, as well as representatives of funding agencies whether public or private, become discouraged, or "turned off," by witnessing the inefficient use of resources. A comprehensive, integrated, and coordinated program will be well received by the community, and the services included will be more acceptable and used more effectively. Conversely, when services are not well coordinated and "patch-work" in nature, they will not be as readily accepted and used. Thus, a downward spiral is put in process. The underused services do not have the desired impact among the community members and this results in a further decrease in the use and acceptance of the services. Community members, subsequently, may be less likely to accept and use services provided by new programs.

At the same time, disenchantment also occurs among the representatives of the funding agencies. Policymakers do not want to spend their money if positive results cannot be readily observed and reported to those who maintain the purse strings or, in the case of private organizations, the donors. In the latter instance, it is not infrequent that progress reports complete with appropriate pictures of success stories are presented to donors and potential donors in order to maintain their financial interest and largesse. When legislative bodies control the public purse strings, they must be convinced that the so-called bang for the buck justifies continued or increased funding.

Disenchantment or discouragement resulting from the lack of coordinated program development is the proverbial double-edged sword. The program's impact in the community is lower resulting in discouragement among community leaders and members. This, in turn, results in a lack of enthusiasm for seeking out or participating in new programs. Also, disenchantment and discouragement among funding sources that observe unacceptably low impact and participation results in a decreased enthusiasm and support for additional or new funding.

REMEDYING THE PROBLEMS

As noted earlier, these problems are neither new nor unknown. Various approaches have been attempted to address them in the past within the Cherokee Nation and among other Indian tribes and communities. The most common approaches involved (1) establishing some type of planning board, (2) allowing the public/private sector to assume control, and (3) doing nothing specific but simply trying to make the best of it. Each approach met with varying levels of success or failure in the past. The Cherokee Nation has tried each approach and various combinations of the approaches at one time or another. However, none was shown to be completely successful in the situations facing the Nation. Given this realization, the Nation sought an innovative approach for coordinating services and programs provided by the public and private sectors. An approach was sought that focused primarily on the process rather than on structural controls. Queries were made of Native American and federal government leaders and representatives, as well as those of private foundations, in hopes of identifying an appropriate and effective strategy for coordination.

One of the more intriguing concepts encountered in the search was the Negotiated Investment Strategy (Strategy). The Strategy was based upon principles of mediation rather than arbitration or control. And it had been tested in three urban areas of the United States (discussed later in the chapter), though never in a rural setting. In any event, the Strategy seemed to be effective when the following conditions prevailed:

(a) there were many parties coexisting in actual or potential conflict;
(b) the need to avoid or resolve the conflict was strong;
(c) the parities involved could be motivated to act and react in a timely fashion; and
(d) the authority for committing the resources necessary for resolving the conflict was in the hands of the participants themselves.

In the eyes of the leaders of the Cherokee Nation of Oklahoma, this was a veritable description of the situations as it existed in northeastern Oklahoma. After learning more about the details and processes related to the Strategy, the Nation's leaders assumed the role of facilitators in order to familiarize the Nation's communities with it and to promote its application locally. Presented here are a brief description of the Strategy's principles and processes, a description of its application among the Cherokee Nation of Oklahoma, and a summary of the results of these efforts.

THE NEGOTIATED INVESTMENT STRATEGY

The Strategy goes beyond the simple principle of citizen participation in programs that are intended to serve them. Earlier works have described models that have been implemented for citizen participation. For example, the "elitist" model exists in which community members serve on boards. The primary purposes of the member participation are fund raising, public relations, and image building (Stanton 1970). In the "advisory" model of citizen participation, community members also serve on boards. In contrast to the elitist model, however, these boards exercise limited powers over policy issues. A third model is the "consumer control" model. Again, the basis for citizen participation is the board. Only in this model, the governing board is dominated by a cross section of community residents. All these models provide only a limited role for community members in the planning and implementation of programs and some are based on an assumption of conflict between management and citizens (Holton et al. 1973).

The Negotiated Investment Strategy is considerably different in several important dimensions. There are six key elements to the Strategy:

1. An impartial mediator is selected to serve as a facilitator (and recording secretary) for the proceedings.
2. Negotiating teams are selected for each group.
3. Prior to the teams' engagement in the negotiating process, there is an informal exchange of information between them.
4. The formal process of negotiation involves face-to-face discussions, mediated by the facilitator.
5. The outcome of the negotiations is a written agreement that contains a set of mutually agreed upon commitments.
6. There is public review and adoption/rejection of the agreement and commitment by the public, when the agreement is approved, and specification of the procedures by which subsequent actions will be monitored and evaluated. In the case of public disapproval, the negotiating teams return to the table for further discussion and resolution of problems responsible for the rejection. In other words, the strategy has a built-in mechanism for iteration rather than termination.

The Value of Negotiation

There is a substantial body of research dealing with and supporting the process of resolving disputes through negotiation (please see, for example, Quirk 1989; Sullivan 1984; Susskind and Cruishank 1989).

Much of the research is based on the premise that negotiation is superior to other methods of conflict/dispute resolution. Quirk (1989) focuses on the "cooperative resolution of conflicts" and points out the gains that can be achieved as a result of "exchanging concessions." Sullivan (1984) suggests that negotiations are ubiquitous in conflicts and disputes and that "reciprocal back scratching beats the contortions necessary for self-sufficiency." Sullivan's approach is based on exchange theory as it emphasizes that those individuals and groups "choose to negotiate when the benefits from the negotiation exceed the cost." In each of the above instances, the primary focus is on settling disputes and resolving conflicts. The starting point of the process, therefore, is the existence of a conflict. In contrast, for the Cherokee Nation of Oklahoma, the central issue and starting point was not a conflict or the need for resolution of a dispute, rather it was a need to build a consensus within the community to in order to avoid a conflict and to ensure integration and coordination.

The work by Susskind and Cruishank (1989) is perhaps the most relevant and pertinent to the concerns of the Cherokee Nation. Though this work, too, is organized around the theme of settling disputes, the process suggested and emphasized is that of consensus building. In line with the principles of the Negotiated Investment Strategy, they point out that this process requires "informal, face to face interaction among representatives of stakeholders," which may appear to be "deceptively simple" but in actuality is an "extraordinarily complex" process. Another point made by Susskind and Cruishank, which pertains to the Cherokee Nation perspective, is the need to "argue not for political compromise, but for voluntary agreements that offer the wisest, fairest, most efficient, and most stable outcomes possible."

Derived from the research discussed above are five perquisites for successful negotiation. (1) The key players must be identified and persuaded that it is in their best interests to sit down and negotiate. (2) Power relationships between the parties must be balanced so that no one party holds an advantage in power. (3) A legitimate spokesperson for each group must be identified and included. (4) The time frame for negotiations and deadlines for reaching an agreement must be realistic. (5) Finally, the dispute must be framed so that it does not violate the basic value of the members of either party entering into negotiation.

PREVIOUS ATTEMPTS AT THE NEGOTIATED INVESTMENT STRATEGY

As mentioned earlier, the Strategy was implemented in three Midwest cities. They included Gary, Indiana; Columbus, Ohio; and, St. Paul, Minnesota. The Federal Regional Council of Chicago, a consortium of representatives from federal programs, sponsored the demonstration projects. Subsequent to these favorable experiences, the state of Connecticut used the Strategy to develop procedures for allocating declining federal funds during the early 1980s. In each of these instances, the ability of the projects to meet their goals was assessed by the Kettering Foundation and the Federal Regional Councils. The study concluded that:

(1) the Strategy effectively expedited intergovernmental agreements in complex developmental projects;

(2) the process itself enhanced the ability to attract and secure private commitments to social development;

(3) both those providing services and those receiving them felt that the Strategy resulted in a more efficient and effective delivery of services; and,

(4) the Strategy was clearly responsible for the resolution of many policy and program conflicts that had been lingering for years.

All parties involved in the use of the Negotiated Investment Strategy felt that it made a significant contribution to the success of the conflict resolution and, ultimately, to the success of their programs. Many participants spoke of the intangible benefits of the process, such as the "personalizing" of intergovernmental relationships and the establishment of communication that had been nonexistent, diminished, or ineffective. This increased communication, in turn, led to better understanding by each party of the other side's constraints, restraints, and abilities.

The Strategy was not without its difficulties, however. The difficulties encountered related to the implementation of the negotiated agreements. It must be kept in mind that there are no legal statutes or compulsions that can be used to sustain the commitments of either party, and there is always the possibility that exogenous events, such as changes in public administrations, funding amounts, or priorities, may occur. Therefore, implementation is always potentially problematic and heavily dependent upon the commitments of individuals rather than organizations. Moreover, the problem of inertia was evident in some instances. There was a tendency to go back to "business as usual" and usually resulted in the subjugation of the Strategy to previous methods.

THE STRATEGY IN THE CHEROKEE NATION

Aware of both the advantages and limitations of the Negotiated Investment Strategy and the fact that it had not been attempted in a rural setting, the Cherokee Nation decided to adopt it. The Strategy was initiated in 1980 when officials from the Cherokee Nation approached the Charles F. Kettering Foundation of Dayton, Ohio, for information and assistance. The Foundation had supported most of the earlier work pertaining to the Strategy and had both the staff to provide the necessary technical assistance and an interest in the proposed project within the Cherokee Nation. The Nation's project was eventually co-sponsored by the U.S. Department of Agriculture (Office of Rural Development Policy) and the Office of Management and Budget.

The Nation's leadership invited the Kettering Foundation staff to eastern Oklahoma to present the concept of the Negotiated Investment Strategy to community leaders from the three counties comprising the majority of the Cherokee Nation population. Also, exploratory meetings were held between the Cherokee Nation and representatives of local governments in the area, in particular mayors and county commissioners. Initially, there was apprehension on both sides. On the part of the Cherokee Nation there was apprehension about prejudice against Native Americans. On the part of the local representatives, there was apprehension that the Cherokee Nation would dominate the Negotiated Strategy process. These apprehensions were overcome through the initial meetings, due in part to the expectation of considerable benefits from the Strategy to be gained by each party to the process.

Ground Rules

A basic set of five "ground rules" was established for the project.

(1) The agenda of items to be negotiated had to be recognized as legitimate by all parties involved.

(2) The negotiating teams had to be comprised of as many individuals as necessary in order to be able to address the full range
of issues determined to be pertinent.

(3) Each team had to have obtained the necessary authority to make
commitments for the group(s) they represented in negotiation.

(4) The negotiating session mediator/facilitator would coordinate
the flow of information and documents between the negotiating teams.

(5) The time frame agreed upon had to be sufficient to reflect the
complexity of the issues to be negotiated but also had to be
brief in order to avoid frustration with the negotiating process.

Selecting the Teams

Three groups or teams of negotiators were identified as necessary to
developing a Negotiated Investment Strategy. These included a team
from the Cherokee Nation of Oklahoma, a team representing the state
of Oklahoma, and a team representing several federal departments and
agencies concerned with projects in the Nation.

The Cherokee group included staff from the Nation and local public officials and community leaders from three counties in Oklahoma
(Adair, Cherokee, and Sequoyah). The three counties are located in
the northeastern part of Oklahoma, near the border with Arkansas. The
majority of the Cherokee Nation's population lives here, and Cherokee
constitute a majority of the population in each county. According to the
1990 U.S. Census, the total population of the three counties was about
56,300 people, of which about 26,500 or 47 percent were Cherokee.
The Cherokee comprise about 44 percent of the total population in Adair
County, 33 percent in Cherokee County, and 21 percent in Sequoyah
County. Prior to Oklahoma statehood (1907), the counties comprised
part of the entry way into the old Indian Territory, and therefore many
residents trace their ancestry to the Cherokee Tribal Rolls.

In 1994 the three counties were part of the Tahlequah Service Unit
of the Oklahoma City Area Indian Health Service (Cameron 1995).
They had large pockets of poverty, substantial levels of unemployment,
and a series of health and other socioeconomic problems. Efforts to
resolve these conditions were complicated by the fragmented and duplica-

tive nature of the services provided to the Cherokee Nation by the federal government (through the Bureau of Indian Affairs), the state of Oklahoma, the three county governments, and the eighteen cities and towns within them. In addition to problems associated with the lack of coordination between these programs, there were serious problems associated with the jurisdiction or "turf" of the various governmental agencies and the differing regulatory constraints of the federal, state, and local governments.

The federal group of negotiators included members of the Federal Regional Councils, the Department of Agriculture, the Office of Management and Budget, and the Bureau of Indian Affairs including the Indian Health Service. The Oklahoma group was comprised of representatives from the Departments of Health and Social Services.

Early Concerns `

Two concerns emerged near the beginning of the project. First, there was concern that all parties with a "substantial stake" in the process and issues would not participate. This concern was directed primarily at the constitution and participation of the federal team. The second concern, also directed primarily at the federal groups, was that the composition of the groups might not include representatives from some key policymakers.

To remedy these concerns and avoid the potential obstacles involved, consideration was given in the earliest days of the project to devising a strategy to convince the potential participants from the federal government (interestingly, primarily the Bureau of Indian Affairs) of the importance of the project. They needed to be convinced of the importance of contributing the time and effort necessary for the project to be successful.

In brief, the strategy was to begin the process with a series of meetings within the three target counties. The purpose was twofold. First, the meetings would educate local people about the idea and its related concepts, and second, they would develop an agenda of concerns from the local perspective. The underlying assumption was that it would be easier to gain the interest of federal officials if they knew which issues concerned the local community teams. In that way, the federal agencies would not be asked to respond in the abstract but rather to the actual concerns expressed by the members of the local community.

Setting a Local Agenda

A series of meetings between the Cherokee Nation group and the local communities was held to develop the local agenda. The first meeting involved a representative group of local officials and community leaders from communities/counties within which the Nation is located and the representatives of the Cherokee Nation. The officials and community leaders were invited to a one-day conference at a university located in Tahlequah, site of the Nation's capital. Representatives from federal rural development agencies also attended. The conference addressed the question: "What are the needs, problems, and opportunities facing the counties and the Nation.

The conference agenda included:

A presentation on the Negotiated Investment Strategy process by the Kettering Foundation and Nation officials;

Small group meetings to generate ideas for priority assignment;

Development of a comprehensive list of local agenda items by group leaders; and,

Plenary group discussion of the comprehensive list, with subsequent voting on priorities.

With assistance from experts in group process and rural development, the meeting identified and developed an initial priority listing for some 130 issues. These issues were grouped into broad categories including water, solid waste, education, economic development, human services, transportation, and public finance. The meeting also produced a list of five issues pertaining to human services concerns. These included the following.

(1) The need to integrate services, that is, to coordinate and possibly consolidate some of the services being provided by the state of Oklahoma, the counties, and the Cherokee Nation.

(2) There was a need to develop a better system for assessing and addressing the health needs of all the rural residents of northeastern Oklahoma.

(3) There was a need to improve the social services delivery system for residents of northeastern Oklahoma, in particular the services relating to welfare of children in the area.

(4) Improvements were needed in the administrative efficiency of the state and federal reimbursement system for therapeutic medical care services. This concern focused on the methods by which providers were being reimbursed for services from Medicaid, Medicare, and Indian Health Services' Contract Care programs.

(5) There was a need for job training programs among the unemployed and underemployed in the region. In particular there was a need for the development of local residents for employment in the health care system.

A second large group meeting was held two months later, attended by representatives of the Cherokee Nation and the county governments in the three-county region. The meeting was held to address the ongoing activities related to the Strategy, to discuss further specific experiences with the Strategy, to re-examine and redefine the priority list derived from the first meeting, and importantly, to determine the composition of the local Strategy negotiating team.

Following this meeting, local groups met on a monthly basis for over a period of one year to further clarify issues. During these meetings, many issues were determined to be of significance to only a portion of the three-county region and/or identified as not requiring formal negotiation. These issues were removed from the list.

At the end of the one-year period, the local representatives reconvened to finalize the agenda. It was determined that almost all issues remaining for consideration required further study to better articulate local area problems and the range of possible remedies. This activity was also viewed as necessary in order to provide adequate justification for federal and/or state assistance. Technical assistance funds were sought for studies in the priority areas of economic development, human services, transportation, public finance, water development, solid waste, and education.

Two members from each of the local teams were selected to represent the participating county or tribe on a "core team." The core team would be the negotiating team representing the local concerns agreed upon by county and Nation representatives. The team composition and its members were selected according to the following criteria:

Official status within the county and Nation's governments;
Private sector representation;
Knowledge of high priority issues;
Power to represent and negotiate concerning high priority issues; and,
Relationship to (degree affected by) high priority concerns.

Thus, the core team represented both the local public and private sectors and served to make Strategy policy decisions for the local area as a whole (in consultation with other local representatives and consultants on specific issues).

Having identified the issues for discussion and the teams that would negotiate with the state and federal teams, the local communities then selected a group to represent it at the negotiations. Members were drawn from persons interested in economic development, health services management, education, transportation, and public health. The attempt here was to develop a membership that would be knowledgeable across a broad spectrum of services needed for a comprehensive solution to the issues identified for negotiation. The local negotiating team included public officials as well as representatives of the private sector interests. Wilma Mankiller, then Deputy Chief of the Cherokee Nation led the team.

The Mediator

The selection of the mediator was deemed critical to the success of the application of the Negotiated Investment Strategy in Oklahoma. The selection was facilitated by the departure from the Kettering Foundation of its representative to the Oklahoma project. (He left to become president of a northeastern university and, therefore, was free from any restrictions associated with employment by the Foundation.) He had been widely praised for his understanding of the negotiating process and his extensive efforts to maintain its momentum in Oklahoma. In 1984 he accepted the request to serve as mediator. It was only at this point in time, with the issues determined from the local perspective and

a mediator agreed upon and agreeing to participate, that the local negotiating team felt confident that it could engage effectively the state and
federal governments in the process.

The Vagaries of Federal Involvement

Each project based on implementing a Negotiated Investment Strategy will deal with a unique set of factors. Nevertheless, it is instructive
to describe here the vagaries that obtained in the Oklahoma project in
terms of dealing with the federal government. They reflect both the
hazards of dealing with government agencies at all levels as well as the
need for persistence and patience on the part of the local communities
and partners.

Initially, securing federal involvement was relatively simple. Members
of the administration in place were familiar with the Negotiated Investment Strategy. In fact it was consistent with other initiatives of the
administration pertaining to such issues as development of a national
urban policy. Therefore, there already existed an organizational framework within which the participation of the Federal Regional Council in
Chicago could be managed. The support of the administration was
pledged and implemented through the Assistant to the President for
Intergovernmental Affairs.

However, the vagaries of dealing with federal administrations
became evident when the federal administrators initially involved were
voted out of office. The incoming administration was even more philo-
sophically supportive of local initiatives such as the Negotiated Investment Strategy; however, the change of administrations actually delayed
federal participation for five years. This delay derived from the federal bureaucracy's hesitancy to become involved in new initiatives
prior to the administration's appointees to each agency making clear
their philosophies and programs. Concomitantly, the local team as
well as the Foundation officials needed time to familiarize the new officials with the proposed project and to educate them as to its potential.
This process was delayed because with the reorganization, reduction,
and elimination of some federal programs, it was not clear just what
departments would be relevant and who the key actors would be for
a federal team.

In the middle of the new administration's first term, high-level support for the Strategy was obtained at the White House level. By then, though, the administration had disbanded the Federal Regional Councils. Thus, their involvement was lost. About one year later the process seemed to coalesce once again as the White House, the Department of Agriculture, and the Office of Management and Budget all publicly indicated support for the project. This notion was made even stronger when both the latter agencies set aside funds to support the process. Subsequently, briefings were held over the period of six months as to what agencies and what representatives of those agencies would comprise the federal team. Finally, four years from the outset in the local communities, the federal team was involved in the first round of negotiations.

The time frame for the entire process was set back considerably by the change in administration and the slow turning of the wheels of bureaucracy. However, one of the ground rules for the Strategy mentioned earlier was successfully met. It is believed essential to the negotiating process that it should be adequate but minimal. In other words, the negotiating process should not be drawn out to the point of reducing interest in or the value of the project. The project complied with this ground rule. Within one and one-half years of the first meeting with the federal government's negotiating team, the meetings were completed, and the recommendations and outcomes were compiled and published.

The State

It is obvious from the description of the Strategy thus far that the Cherokee Nation and residents of the three target counties were the motivating and sustaining forces in the effort to use the Strategy as a medium for developing a seamless, coordinated approach to economic and social development. The state of Oklahoma was very pleased with the concept and development of the project in its initial stages but decided on a reactive rather than a proactive involvement in the ongoing process during its early stages of development. While the reasons behind the state's apparent ambivalence were never made explicit, some informed speculations can be made.

The state of Oklahoma has some seventy-seven county governments and populations with which to deal. Some state officials might have been concerned about how the remaining counties would view the state's entering into the rather sophisticated and complex negotiating process with three counties. There may also have been concern that the negotiations would lead to a disproportionately large share of the state's resources being funneled to the three counties.

There was some concern expressed among state officials as to what precedents might be set in the process. Would each or various groups of counties, in the future, demand similar strategies and engage in strategic negotiations pertaining to every problem and issue facing them? What impact would this have in terms of the number of state personnel necessary in each situation? Would agencies and representatives be overwhelmed by a wide-scale adoption of the process? What would be the complications inherent in trying to devise a specific solution to common problems occurring across the state?

Finally, there might have been some concern on the part of the state that the negotiating process, which includes the individual assessment of problems affecting local populations, would lead to the "resurrection" of controversial issues, such as water management, that the state felt had already been "resolved."

In any event, the state maintained a passive role in the long run, up to the actual stage of negotiation when federal funding became available to support the process. At that time, the state joined in with considerable enthusiasm and good faith. State officials gave two reasons for their enthusiasm. First, they felt that the state would be able to maintain power sufficient to minimize or limit any negative outcomes that might occur with regard to earlier trepidation about the negotiating process mentioned above. Second, they expressed an apparent real and sincere interest in working closer with the Cherokee Nation. It should also be mentioned that by this time, the Nation had received considerable national attention for its attempts at creative approaches to economic, health, and social development. And in addition, the state's position with regard the new federal policies had changed, and it had added responsibilities in terms of handling problems locally. Meanwhile, the Nation had kept a "safe distance" from the state by maintaining its independence. In fact, the negotiation process itself contributed to an even greater sense of independence in the Nation.

REFLECTIONS ON THE DEVELOPMENTAL PROCESS

After several years marked by alternating periods of setbacks and progress, the mechanisms and actors were in place for the actual negotiations to begin. It is instructive to provide a retrospect on this phase of the process. Three major issues are considered important namely, bringing people to the negotiating table, alterating the traditional power structure, and being willing to acknowledge the "power" of each participant and their commitment.

The Issues

What brought the agencies and their representatives into the process and, ultimately, to the negotiating table? Obviously, each group participated in the process for different reasons. From the federal perspective, for example, officials were working within a new philosophical framework within which more local solutions to local problems were encouraged. Moreover, federal officials saw an opportunity for an innovative approach to the resolution of problems longstanding in rural areas. They recognized that, despite the seemingly disproportionate amount of time and resources spent in dealing with problems of rural America, insufficient progress was being made. This was especially true, for example, in the area of health service delivery, wherein over the past decades, several large-scale programmatic efforts to improve the rural health system had been substantially less than completely successful. There was also recognition that federal departments were often devoting resources to rural policy issues beyond their legislative mandate. For instance, the Department of Agriculture found itself occasionally involved in issues, such as health, that were perceived as only tangentially related to agriculture. Thus, federal departments and agencies were willing to participate in an experimental program that might lead to an appropriate reduction in their responsibility.

State officials "wanted" to participate out of recognition that they bear significant responsibilities for the economic and social needs of all Oklahoma residents, including those in northeastern Oklahoma. Moreover, under the new federal philosophy and funding mechanisms (such as block grants), the state was expected by the federal government, and increasingly by its residents, to take even greater responsibility and accountability for development and funding local programs. Thus, there was the added incentive that, whatever the drawbacks, the Negotiated Investment Strategy would contribute to a more efficient and responsible use of financial resources. It became clear that the state saw the need for a new strategy to replace the traditionally ineffective and inefficient approach to resolving problems identified by Oklahomans.

Finally, the inspiration for the local team was quite clear. The Strategy was certainly in its self-interest. It was a professional and effective way to express their needs. By engaging state and federal officials in a mutually agreed upon process, the local representatives were positioned in such a way that they could not be ignored. It was also recognized, and indeed was the basis for development of the Strategy, that it had a high probability of reducing inefficiencies and other problems pertaining to the traditionally fragmented, uncoordinated, and duplicative approach to solving local problems. Also, through participation in the Strategy the local agencies and their representative gained "status" in terms of their dealings with both state and dederal officials. Finally, the Strategy allowed the local representatives to identify and develop priorities for addressing local problems.

The Strategy

Some of the same reasoning discussed above is pertinent to the issue of why these "power groups" would be willing to share their power with others or perhaps even negotiate away some of those powers. Both state and federal officials acknowledged that, even though they did in fact hold the ultimate regulatory and fiscal authorities, they could not use those powers effectively without local participation. In simple terms, it was a matter of realizing that whether or not they met their mandated and moral responsibilities would depend on the local people. Given the period within which this Strategy was developed, the political and administrative incentives were obvious. The federal philosophy of returning power and responsibility to the states was in place. Block grant funding meant a reduction in total allotment to the states as well as increased responsibility transferred to the states for determining the priority of problems and funding. Therefore, the states found themselves with considerably more responsibility and often with fewer fiscal resources than previously. It was obvious that it was also in their self-interest to consider and at least experiment with the Negotiated Investment Strategy as an effective mechanism.

The Investment

It is apparent from the foregoing discussion that patience and commitment are necessary and vital elements in the Negotiated Investment Strategy. Moreover, these elements are not uniformly distributed among the participating groups. At the local level, the patience and commitment to the process was exceptionally high. At times, however, the level of patience demonstrated might have actually worked against development of the process. Rather than patiently enduring delays at almost every turn from the state and federal representatives, the local interests and the process itself might have been better served with a more forthright response.

Though initially reticent, once the state came "on board" (no doubt prompted by changes in the federal funding philosophy), it took a very sincere, active, and supportive role in the process. Finally, the greatest difficulty came with gaining the final commitment to the Strategy from the federal level. This could be attributed to a number of reasons discussed earlier including the inertia of bureaucracy in resisting change and the tendency of federal departments and agencies to defend the mandate and funding responsibilities legislated to each.

In summary, the patience and especially the level of commitment to the process displayed by the parties seemed to vary inversely with the size of the bureaucracy involved and distance from the local community. Local representatives seemed to have inordinate levels of patience and commitment to the process. On the one hand, at times the patience demonstrated seemed beyond reason. However, without it the process probably would have failed. This is a caution to those local agencies and their representatives considering engaging in the process.

The Negotiations

The first comprehensive Strategy session involving local, state, and federal negotiating teams occurred four years after the Cherokee Nation made its initial inquiry about the Negotiated Investment Strategy to the Kettering Foundation. The meeting took place at Cherokee Nation headquarters in Tahlequah, with the local team as host. Team leaders met the evening before the session to confirm the agenda and ground rules. Among the ground rules, it was established and agreed upon that:

> The team leader was designated as the spokesperson for the team;
> There would be no audio recording;
> Videotaping would be limited and used later for instructional purposes only;
> Decisions by each team would be made by any process agreed upon by that team;
> Decisions derived from the negotiating session would be based upon a consensus of all three teams;
> Teams could caucus at any time upon request;
> Decisions made in the session would be recorded by the mediator and would be subject to final review and acceptance by team leaders; and, finally,
> It was decided that, should it be necessary as the negotiating process proceeded, the ground rules could be modified by consensus of all three teams.

It is instructive to list the agenda for the first comprehensive Negotiated Investment Strategy session. Major items on the agenda included:

> Presentation of an overview of the Strategy, including a presentation by the mediator on the process and on the initial ground rules that had been agreed upon;
> A presentation on the demographics of the target populations of northeastern Oklahoma;
> Presentations by each team outlining what it expected from the Strategy process;
> Opportunity for each team to present issues (both the federal and state teams chose not to present issues, reserving the right to do so at a later date. The local team presented thirty-two issues

organized into seven categories. Federal team members had been sent a briefing book containing executive summaries of the economic development, education, health and human services, local finance, and waste management studies conducted by the local teams); and,

Planning for the second session, including communication meetings and location, date, and time.

First Session Results

Decisions resulting from the first session affected each of the negotiating teams. For example, the local team was expected to:

Prepare more comprehensive discussion papers on each of the issues identified; and,

Answer the following questions:

What are the barriers to achieving the desired solutions to the problems identified without engaging in the Negotiated Strategy Investment process?

Where would "new" money be involved in the proposed solutions to those problems identified? and,

Would there be additional agencies that ought to be brought into the process to resolve the issue/problem?

The state team was asked and agreed to respond to the issues raised by the local team. The state agreed to:

Prepare a listing of state expenditures in the three-county area that relate to issues presented by the local team;

Consult with the local team on state enterprise zone legislation;

Discuss with the local team:

The applicability of legislation in regard to research on student achievement;

The need for a three-county school improvement program;

The applicability of legislation with regard to research on student achievement;

The development of a rural-based model of obstetric care;

A cooperative pilot project to reduce duplication in the provision of health care services;

The possibility of arranging discussions between state job-training professionals and the Cherokee Nation;

The need for community-based care for the disabled and mentally retarded; and,

The possibility of using a mini-form of the Strategy to provide local public input to state health and human services priorities.

The federal team agreed to:

Prepare a response to the local proposal for the development of a comprehensive water plan; and,

Provide requested information to the Cherokee Nation Department of Education.

In addition, it was decided that subgroups of teams could meet between Strategy sessions to clarify issues, reach agreement on issues, and determine implementation procedures. Further, it was agreed that subgroups could meet with only two teams represented if it were determined and agreed that the third team was not involved in the issue under discussion. However, all agreements made with only two groups represented were subject to approval by the three teams at the next full Strategy session. All agreements and/or disagreements derived from such meetings would be reported to the facilitator/mediator for use in planning the subsequent session.

Many participants in the first session felt that, while useful, it did not meet with their prior expectations. In assessing the reasons for this, participants identified several pertinent items, which may have reflected the inexperience of each team with the Strategy process. For example, the federal team reportedly began the discussion by stating that no program funds were available. This point struck the local and state teams as irrelevant since from their point of view new funds were not a major issue. Thus, the statement set a negative tone for the meeting. Moreover, not all members of the federal team knew one another, and some were not familiar with the Strategy process and/or the local agenda. Finally, the federal team came to the table with no issues to present. Again, these facts contributed to creation of a less than positive atmosphere for negotiations.

The local team failed to provide sufficient explanation and documentation to the federal and state teams concerning the local issues. With the exception of executive summaries, additional information was provided only on the day of the meeting.

Finally, the initial state involvement, as noted earlier, was largely to show good faith they brought no specific issues to the table for negotiation.

The Second Session

Several months after the first session, a second meeting was held in Tulsa, hosted by the state team. More substantive discussions were held at this meeting. The agenda for the second session included:

Meetings of individual subgroups on specific issues;

Reports by the local, state, and federal teams on their intersession activities including which issues could be eliminated either because they had been resolved, were no longer of concern to the team that proposed them, or were beyond the scope of the Strategy process;

Suggestion of additional issues;

Setting time limits for completing the Negotiated Investment Strategy process; and,

The implementation process.

Results of the second strategy session included the elimination of six issues. Three were resolved, two were found to be beyond the scope of the Strategy process, and one was solved outside the Strategy process. Progress was reported on four issues, and four new issues were added. Importantly, two issues were added by the federal team, and this reflected a greater involvement and more active interest on the part the federal government agencies involved.

In addition to these actions it was decided that each of the subgroups would prepare and submit a proper record of all decisions made to date and the resolutions achieved. And each team was to organize a process to eliminate specific issues by the next session. This would involve the development of an "action" agenda that would identify the individuals responsible for the proposed actions on each issue. Two months later the local teams had prepared and disseminated the action agenda.

APPLYING THE STRATEGY: LESSONS LEARNED

One of the most important insights gained from the experience of initiating, developing, and finally completing the Negotiated Investment Strategy was an understanding of the importance of identifying, encouraging, and bringing to the table all the key actors. There is no small price to pay if someone or some agency ends up not being invited to participate. Discussions are necessarily limited and, most importantly, final compromises and commitments are hampered and reduced in effectiveness. A corollary to this lesson is that it is essential to identify, as nearly as possible, the full complement of issues and nuances of each problem being addressed. Without this step, the identification of appropriate participants cannot be completed.

And it is very important that the issues be made relevant to each of the participants. This means ensuring that the issue is viewed from the perspective of each vested interest. The potential benefits as well as costs that accrue to each participant should be annunciated and estimated. When possible, bottom line cost-benefit analyses should be attempted.

Timing is very important. First, adequate but not an excessive amount of time must be allowed for local participants to develop a full understanding of the issues, their meaning to the community, and the priority that should be placed on each. Also, they must be educated on their own influence, or power, within the political process. In the past, many Indian communities have adopted a "reservation mentality" and have quietly accepted those programs deemed "necessary and appropriate" by federal and state officials. One of the barriers to full and enthusiastic participation at the local level is the feeling that nothing can be done to change this situation. And, moreover, attempts to change the system might result in penalties, such as reduced consideration of important issues and an associated reduction in financial resources to address local problems. Therefore, the time devoted to building both a sense of mission and confidence among the local people is vital and must be adequate.

It is also important to examine what are often complex problems on an issue-by-issue basis. Thus, it is necessary for the local leadership not only to be fully informed about a problem raised by the members of the community but also to be able to "dissect" it into the pertinent issues or elements. By doing this, the necessary local actors can be identified and brought into the process. Far more can be achieved in this manner when the sectors identified integrate their strategic and programmatic thinking. Greater success was achieved when the issues were "tied into tidy bundles" by location, sector, and "problem."

There was a consensus among the larger players involved that one of the strengths of the Negotiated Investment Strategy was that it was a singular situation. In other words, at the state and federal levels there was a feeling that the success achieved was due at least in part to the "uniqueness" of the Strategy. There was some belief that the process would be cumbersome and difficult to manage if applied more generally. There was concern at the state and federal levels, as well as at the local level, that if the process or any part of the process were to be institutionalized, it would probably lose much of its value.

However, at the same time, there was support for putting in place a mechanism for referring to and using the Strategy on an as needed basis. This was particularly the case at the local level. It was also believed, especially in rural areas, that a small staff should be developed to oversee and monitor the process when activated. This reflects the fact that rural programs are generally understaffed and the recognition that an activity such as the Strategy requires individuals dedicated to it. In turn, this points to the need for some source of funding at the local, state, and federal levels to support local Strategy efforts.

Finally, and this returns to some of the issues raised above, the pre-negotiation processes are probably at least as important as any other stage in the Negotiated Investment Strategy. For example, during the team-building period, it is important to build a consensus among the local participants regarding the identification of the relevant issues. Moreover, it is important for the team to achieve a consensus and present a concordant position in the negotiating sessions. To do this, the local team and its members must achieve and express confidence in the concerns identified and the belief that necessary change is likely to result from the negotiations.

GENERALIZING THE EXPERIENCE

The Negotiated Investment Strategy, by dint of its specificity in terms of problems addressed, the environment in which the process takes place, and the actors identified to participate in the process will be unique to each situation. Nevertheless, there are a number of reasons why the process itself can be utilized in other areas. The Oklahoma Negotiated Investment Strategy was an experiment. It marked the first time that the process had been attempted in a rural area. The experience of the Cherokee Nation of Oklahoma suggests that the Strategy can be used successfully in other rural areas. Participants described several positive results that are pertinent to other efforts.

(1) The Negotiated Investment Strategy brought people together in a positive and constructive manner. Local people from small communities distributed across a rather large rural area communicated, often for the first time, about mutual problems. Thus, at this level, a greater sense of solidarity was achieved, which was important not only in addressing the immediate problem but in setting the stage for continued collaboration on other problems as well.

In addition, groups that in the past may have experienced contacts that could be described as confrontational, agreed that these meetings were characterized by collaboration and a mutual concern to reach positive conclusions that would benefit all parties involved.

(2) The Negotiated Investment Strategy helped to demonstrate and focus (or in some instances, refocus) participants' attention (at both the individual and agency level) on the multiple dimensions of significant policy issues. This was especially true in the areas of health and education. In the process of considering these issues and their components, linkages between the sectors were revealed. In turn, the need for closer cooperation was demonstrated and, importantly, accepted.

(3) The Negotiated Investment Strategy resulted in a greater coordination of efforts and was therefore the better use of limited resources beyond the problems originally considered for negotiation. For example, within the Cherokee Nation of Oklahoma the Strategy resulted in a much higher degree of coordination. Also, there are increased levels of coordination of strategic and operating plans involving the Departments of Health and Social Services at the state level on the one hand and the Cherokee Nation on the other. Representatives of each group/ agency meet annually and jointly coordinate one another's plans in the areas of health, social, and economic programs and services. Differ-

ences that emerge are negotiated. Thus, the funds made available from the state of Oklahoma and those from the Indian Health Service are put to the most effective and efficient use by minimizing unnecessary overlap and duplication. There is a consensus that the negotiated process leads to maximizing the potential returns from the various sources of financing.

(4) The Negotiated Investment Strategy leads to more effective programs. Coupled with the increased coordination and planning among participants, there is the impression that programs are more effective now than prior to use of the Negotiated Investment Strategy. While the evidence to date is anecdotal, there is a feeling among the local communities that the target populations more readily accept solutions to problems identified locally and developed locally. Here, reference should be made to the previous chapter on self-help, wherein the need for communities to identify with or "own" a problem and its solution are important to success.

(5) The Negotiated Investment Strategy experience has led to positive changes in the ability of the various programs as well as the Cherokee Nation of Oklahoma to respond to current issues. There is a strong feeling that the inertia of negative bureaucratic administrative procedures has been reduced through the process and agencies and organizations are more willing to consider alternative, community based initiatives regarding the identification and resolution of problems.

On the basis of the Cherokee Nation's experience and the experiences of other locations with the Strategy, it is evident that the process is likely to be useful when:

> There is a legitimate agenda;
> The number, interests, and expertise of participants/agencies is maximized;
> Authority for committing resources is identified and included in the process;
> Coordination is made a top priority;
> Realistic time limits are placed on the process and parties are motivated to act accordingly.

Also, it is likely that the Strategy process will be more difficult and less cost-effective when:

> Not all parties with a substantial stake in the issues and process are included;
> Those negotiating lack the authority to commit resources;
> At least one party (team, team member) has little intention of working toward a mutually-acceptable outcome;
> One or more of the parties requires time/and or resources beyond those likely to be available for the completion of the process; and,
> One or more parties judge the expenditure of time, energy, and resources to resolve the issue(s) to be unjustified.

Further, rural areas generally face more difficulties than urban areas when considering implementing the Negotiated Investment Strategy. Rural areas generally do not have a single political entity or representative with the power to identify a local team and require adherence to a set schedule. Also, leadership is more diffused in rural settings. The opinions and desires of a broad range of overlapping and sometimes independent governmental units must be considered and brought into the process. In the northeast Oklahoma experience this included, for example, the Cherokee Nation as well town and county governments.

Rural areas are also more likely to be limited in their ability to respond to technical issues or issues that require innovative solutions. Many rural public officials are (more or less) voluntary public servants with other principal occupations. Therefore, they have limited time and/or resources for additional responsibilities associated with the Strategy. Moreover, most small towns and rural communities do not have a pool of professional talent on which to rely for research and/or technical assistance.

Finally, the Negotiated Investment Strategy was designed to place the local area in the decision-making position in dealing with state and federal agencies, the reverse of the traditional situation. Given the lack of concentrated political power and resources in many rural areas, state and federal representatives may be unwilling to abdicate their authority in the decision-making process.

CONCLUSION

The Negotiated Investment Strategy cannot and should not be viewed by Indian communities as a panacea for the frustrations and concerns of uncoordinated, duplicative, inefficient, and ineffective planning. There are problems inherent in the process as described in this chapter and, without the total commitment of the local communities, reaching the stage of negotiation with funding agencies/organizations is problematical. However, once negotiations are engaged, the potential for positive results is considerable. In addition to the direct impact of the Strategy on resolution of problems, there are ancillary benefits as well. Engaging in the process increased the communication between widely scattered Cherokee communities. And participation increased the sense of community and solidarity among the Cherokee of northeastern Oklahoma. This is crucial to the survival and continued renaissance of the Cherokee culture and traditions. Like any other tool, however, the efficacy of the Negotiated Investment Strategy will be determined by the skill with which it is used. The experience of the Cherokee Nation in northeastern Oklahoma bodes well for other Indian communities finding themselves in similar situations.

The Cherokee Experience and Beyond

It was a spirit of survival and perseverance that carried the Cherokee to Indian Territory on the Trail of Tears. Today, it is the same spirit leading the Cherokees on a new trail—the trail of opportunity. Since the earliest contact with the explorers in the 1500s, the Cherokee Nation has been identified as one of the most advanced among Native American tribes. After contact with the European immigrants in the southeastern United States, the Cherokee culture continued to develop, modify, and progress with acquisitions from the European settlers. Without warning, in 1838, thousands of Cherokee men, women, and children were assembled and moved a thousand miles away to Indian Territory in what is today the state of Oklahoma. Hundreds died along the way.

In Indian Territory, the Cherokees soon rebuilt their democratic form of government, churches, schools, newspapers, and businesses. A new constitution was adopted in September of 1839, the year in which the final group of Cherokees arrived on the Trail of Tears. They rebuilt their lifestyle from the remnants of the society and culture that they carried with them to their new homeland. An age of relative prosperity ended with division over the Civil War. Because they had been persuaded to side with the Confederacy during the war, what remained of tribal land was divided into individual allotments that were given to Cherokees listed in the census compiled by the Dawes Commission in the late

1890s. Descendants of those original enrollees make up today's Chero-kee Nation tribal membership.

In 1907, with Oklahoma statehood, the Cherokee Nation was dis-solved. During the twentieth century, the Cherokee have faced repeated attempts to eliminate them as a people and culture. From time to time, these efforts have included federal policies and legislation to relocate them to urban areas and the elimination of their schools and tribal rights. Through it all, the Cherokee have fought to keep their traditions and nation alive.

In 1971, the Cherokee Nation government was reorganized and the first elected chief since Oklahoma statehood was appointed. Today, the federally recognized Cherokee Nation is the second largest Indian tribe in the United States. There are more than 182,000 tribal members. Almost 70,000 Cherokees reside in the 7,000-square-mile area of the Cherokee Nation of Oklahoma. The area is not a reservation but a juris-dictional service area that includes all of eight counties and portions of six counties in northeastern Oklahoma. The area lies within the bound-aries of the historical Cherokee Nation, extant there before the Civil War.

As a federally recognized Indian tribe, the Nation has both the oppor-tunity and the sovereign right to exercise control and development of tribal assets. On February 10, 1990, the Cherokee Nation authorized the negotiation of a tribal self-governance agreement for direct funding from the U.S. Congress. The agreement authorizes the tribe to plan, con-duct, consolidate, and administer programs and receive direct funding to deliver services to tribal members. Self-governance is a change from the paternalistic controls that the federal government has exercised in the past to the full-tribal responsibility for self-government and inde-pendence intended by treaties with sovereign Indian Nations. The self-determination policy encourages tribes to maintain and perpetuate their cultures and heritage. A basic principle of self-determination is a government-to-government relationship. The federal government now deals with tribal governments much the same as it deals with state and local governments.

This self-government and independence is practiced, however, within a special relationship with the federal government. The U.S. govern-ment has responsibility for ensuring the natural and financial resources, which the Secretary of the Interior holds in trust for American Indian

Tribes. And at the same time, the Tribal governments are dependent upon the federal government to provide services directly to tribes under the many treaties, laws, and court decisions that govern Indian affairs.

In spite of the recognition of the principle of Native self-determination and the value of maintaining and perpetuating Native American cultures, Indians must still be alert to threats to their existence and face challenges to the integrity of their tribes. In this book, we have discussed several experiences that demonstrate these threats.

INDIAN IDENTITY

In the late 1980s, for example, there emerged an attempt by the federal government to legislate Indian identity for the purposes of determining eligibility for federally funded health care services. As proposed and described in this volume, the federal legislation would impose criteria for the determination of Indian identity. Moreover, if implemented, the criteria would effectively terminate members of certain groups of Indians, fractionate some Indian families, and deprive some Indians of health services. To many Indians the proposed changes in Indian identity in order to qualify for health services were taken as evidence of a new era of "termination" and another example of "failed federal responsibility." Fortunately, the proposed federally legislated criterion based almost solely on blood quantum was modified prior to the final passage of the Indian Health Care Improvement Act of 1992. Nevertheless, this attempt points up the need for the Indian community to be on guard constantly to protect even their identity.

SELF-HELP

In this volume the issue of self-help within the Cherokee Nation was used to illustrate its value for establishing and nurturing community responsibility for health improvement. But it is also offered as an example of how self-help can be used not only for the purposes of health improvement but in other important areas if community life as well. The ultimate goal here is to demonstrate how the concepts of self-reliance and local control, while providing an effective means of dealing with community problems, can lead to an increased level of solidarity within the Indian community. Moreover, the concept of self-help is compatible with and contributes to the important principle of self-determination within the special relationships established between the federal government and tribal governments.

NEGOTIATED INVESTMENT STRATEGY

Finally, the concept of the Negotiated Investment Strategy has been described and an illustration of its use by the Cherokee Nation presented. Again, the focus has been on how this strategy could be used to more effectively identify health problems facing Indian communities. The Strategy can be used to more effectively develop, organize, integrate, and implement programs aimed at improving the health status of Indian people. The requirements for a successful Strategy are many, and it is not a simple process. Above all else, it seems that the local Indian communities must be totally committed to it. However, the potential payoffs in terms of problem identification and definition and organizational and program integration and coordination are substantial. Another important derivative of the Negotiated Investment Strategy for the Cherokee has been the increased communication within the Nation, the increased solidarity among the communities, and most importantly perhaps, the sense of self-determination and confidence. Self-sufficiency is the mission of the Cherokee Nation tribal government. Under its current leadership, the tribe has been prepared to enter the twenty-first century on its own terms.

LESSONS LEARNED

Initially, this book was undertaken to demonstrate how one tribal group, the Cherokee Nation, approached the problem of threats to health services as well as the inadequate levels of health services and uncoordinated efforts to deal with its health problems. By describing Cherokee Nation experience in dealing with the problems of improving the health services and health status of the people of the community, this book may offer other Indian tribal groups benefits. The Cherokee Nation's experience and that of every Indian tribal group will be unique. Tribal traditions, experience, and environment all contribute to differences from place to place and time to time. Nevertheless, when adapted to individual settings, the concepts of self-help and the Negotiated Investment Strategy should be considered in attempts to resolve health problems facing any Native American group.

The concepts of preservation of self-identity, self-help, and the Negotiated Investment Strategy go beyond application to health issues. They speak directly to the solidarity of Indian tribal groups and their aspirations for solidarity, independence, self-sufficiency, and self-determination. And, by so doing, these concepts and derivative actions can make positive contributions to the continued emergence and perpetuation of Indian culture in the United States.

References

Ambler, M. 1991. Indian energies devoted to self-sufficiency. *National Forum* (spring): 21–23.

American Indian Policy Review Commission Task Force Six. 1976. Report on Indian health: Final report to the American Indian Policy Review Commission. Washington, D.C.: U.S. Government Printing Office.

Anonymous. 1998. Clinton's failure: Health security reform plan of 1993. http://my.netian.com/~pynchon/doc/healthcare.htm.

Bahr, H., B. Chadwick, and R. Day, eds. 1972. *Native Americans today: A sociological perspective*. New York: Harper and Row.´

Bashshur, R. Office of Research and Development, Indian Health Service. 1979. Technology serves the people. Washington, D.C.: GPO.

Bashshur, R., W. Steeler, and T. Murphy. 1987. On changing Indian eligibility for health care. *American Journal of Public Health* 77 (6).

Bennett, Claude F. 1993. Interdependence models. *Journal of Extension*, vol. 31, no. 2. http://www.joe.org.

Boston Women's Health Book Collective. 1973. *Our bodies, ourselves*. New York: Simon and Schuster Publications.

Burnett, J. 1839. *Cherokee Indian removal 1838–39*. Trail of Tears National Historic Trail, Comprehensive Management and Use Plan, U.S. Dept. of Interior, National Park Service.

Burt, L. 1986. Roots of the Native American urban experience: Relocation policy in the 1950s. *American Indian Quarterly* 10 (2):85–99.

Cameron, D. 1995. Statistical profile of the demographic and health status for the Cherokee Nation of Oklahoma. Memorandum to Dr. Gary W. Shannon, from D. Cameron, Director, Statistical Services, Office of Program Planning and Evaluation, Oklahoma City Area Indian Health Service, Department of Health & Human Services, Oklahoma City, Oklahoma.

Carlson, R. 1975. *The end of medicine*. New York: John Wiley & Sons.

Catlin, George. [1841] 1973. *Letters and notes on the manners, customs, and conditions of the North American Indians*. Reprint, New York: Dover.

Cherokee Nation Public Affairs Department. 1997. Mission statement. Tahlequah, Oklahoma.

Coe, Joffre L. 1961. Cherokee Archeology. In *Symposium on Cherokee and Iroquois culture*, ed. W. Fenton, J. Fenton, and J. Gulick. Bureau of American Ethnology, Bulletin 180:51-60. Washington, D.C.: Smithsonian Institution.

Cohen, F. 1971. *Handbook of federal Indian laws*. Albuquerque: University of New Mexico Press.

Corea, E. 1977. *Nonalignment: the dynamics of a movement*. Toronto: Canadian Institute of International Affairs.

Daniels, J. 1992. The Indian population of North America in 1492. *William and Mary Quarterly* 49 (2):298–320.

Department of Health and Human Services. 1991. Healthy people 2000: National health promotion and disease prevention objectives. DHHS Publication No. 91-50212.

Department of Labor. 1995. Negotiated rulemaking. http://www.dol.gov/dol/asp/public/programs/negreg/negbrief.htm.

Ehrenreich, J., and B. Ehrenreich. 1970. *American health empire* [a report from the health policy advisory center]. New York: Random House.

Eschbach, K. 1992. Shifting boundaries: Regional variation in patterns of identification as American Indians. Ph.D. diss., Harvard University.

Fabrega, H. 1973. Toward a model of illness behavior. *Medical Care* 11 (6): 470–84.

Federal Register 51, no. 111 (1986): 21118-22 (42 C.F.R. pt. 36). Indian Health Services: Eligibility.

Federal Register 52, no. 179 (1987): 35044-50 (42 C.F.R. pt. 36). Indian Health Services: Final Rule.

Fleming, G., A. Giachello, R. Anderson, and A. Andrade. 1984. Self-care: Substitute, supplement, or stimulus for formal medical care services? *Medical Care* 22 (10):950–66.

Fogelson, R. 1961. Change, persistence, and accommodation in Cherokee medico-magical beliefs. In *Symposium on Cherokee and Iroquois culture*, ed. W. Fenton, J. Fenton, and J. Gulick. Bureau of American Ethnology, Bulletin 180, no. 21:213–25. Washington, D.C.: Smithsonian Institution.

Fogelson, R., and P. Kutsche. 1961. Cherokee economic cooperatives: The Gadugi. In *Symposium on Cherokee and Iroquois culture*, ed. W. Fenton, J. Fenton, and J. Gulick. Bureau of American Ethnology, Bulletin 180, no. 11:83–123. Washington, D.C.: Smithsonian Institution.

Foreman, G. 1966. *Indian removal: The emigration of the five civilized tribes of Indians*. Norman: University of Oklahoma Press.

Fox, R. 1977. The medicalization of American society. In *Doing better and feeling worse*. J. Knowles, ed. New York: Norton.

Friedson, E. 1970. *Professional dominance: The social structure of medical care*. New York: Atherton.

Friedson, E. 1976. *Doctoring together: A study of professional social control.* New York: Elsevier.

Fuchs, M. 1974. Health care patterns of urbanized Native Americans. Ph.D. diss., University of Michigan.

Gabel, J., H. Cohen, and S. Fink. 1989. Americans' views on health care: Foolish inconsistencies. *Health Affairs* (spring): 103–12.

Gartner, A., and F. Riessman. 1980. Made for each other: Self-help groups and mental health agencies. *Community Mental Health* 13: 28–32.

Gearing, F. 1961. The rise of the Cherokee State as an instance in a class: The Mesopotamian career to statehood. In *Symposium on Cherokee and Iroquois culture*, ed. W. Fenton, and J. Gluck. Bureau of American Ethnology, Bulletin 180, no. 12. Washington, D.C.: Smithsonian Institution.

Goggin, J. 1961. Commentary. In *Symposium on Cherokee and Iroquois culture*, ed. W. Fenton, and J. Gluck. Bureau of American Ethnology, Bulletin 180, no. 12:77–81. Washington, D.C.: Smithsonian Institution.

Goodwyn, L. 1976. *Democratic promise: the populist movement in America.* New York: Oxford University Press.

Gurian, J. 1977. The importance of dependency in Native American-White contact. *American Indian Quarterly* 3 (1):16-36.

Haug, M., and B. Lavin. 1983. *Consumerism in medicine.* Sage Publications: London.

Holton, W., F. New, and R. Hessler. 1973. Citizen participation and conflict. *Administration in Mental Health* (fall): 96–103

Illich, I. 1976. *Limits to medicine: Medical nemesis: The expropriation of health.* New York: Pantheon Books.

Indian Health Service. 1994. *Trends in Indian health: 1994 tables.*

Jorgesen, J. 1969. Indians and the metropolis. *Social Forces* 48:243ff.

Josephy, A. 1968. *The Indian heritage of America.* New York: Knopf.

Katz, A. 1991. Self-help groups and professional: General issues. In *Self-help: Concepts and applications*, ed. H. Katz, C. Hendricks, and C. Koop. Philadelphia: Charles Press.

Katz, A. 1993. *Self-help in America: A social movement perspective.* New York: Twayne Publishers.

Katz, A. and E. Bender. 1976. Self-help groups in Western society: history and prospects. *The Journal of Applied Behavioral Science.* 12(3): 265–82.

Katz, D., and R. Kahn. 1966. *The social psychology of organizations.* New York: John Wiley & Sons.

King, D., ed. 1979. *The Cherokee Indian Nation.* Knoxville: University of Tennessee Press.

Knowles, J. 1977. *Doing better and feeling worse.* New York: Norton.

Kropotkin, P. 1939. *Mutual aid: A factor in evolution.* London: Penguin Books.

Leventhal, G., K. Maton, E. Madara, and M. Julien. 1990. The birth and death of self-help groups: An ecological perspective. In *Helping one another: Self-help groups in a changing world,* ed. A. Katz, and E. Bender. Oakland, California: Third Party Publishers.

Levin, L., A. Katz, and E. Holst. 1976. *Self-care: Lay initiatives in health.* New York: Prodist.

Lieberman, M. 1979. Help-seeking and self-help groups. In *Self-help groups for coping with crisis: Origins, members, processes, and impact.* New York: Jossey-Bass Publishers.

Logan, A. 1988. New eligibility for Indian health services: Notice of proposed rulemaking. Federal Register, 42 C.F.R. pt. 36, subpts. A-C. 100th Congress, Senate Hearing 912: 207.

Lounsbury, F. 1961. Iroquois-Cherokee linguistic relations. In *Symposium on Cherokee and Iroquois culture,* ed. W. Fenton, and J. Gulick, Bureau of American Ethnology, Bulletin 180, no. 3:11–23. Washington, D.C.: Smithsonian Institution.

Lujan, M. 1991. Federal responsibility to the first Americans. *National Forum* (spring): 13–14.

Maslow, A. 1970. *Motivation and personality,* 2d ed. New York: Harper & Row.

McKeown, T. 1979. *The role of medicine: Dream, mirage or nemesis.* Princeton University Press.

McLoughlin, W. 1993. *After the trail of tears: The Cherokees' struggle for sovereignty, 1839–1880.* Chapel Hill, N.C.: University of North Carolina Press.

McLoughlin, W., and W. Conser. 1989. The first man was red: Cherokee responses to the debate over Indian origins, 1760-1860. *American Quarterly* 41:243–64.

Meriam, L., ed. 1928. *The problems of Indian administration.* Baltimore: Johns Hopkins Press, Institute for Government Research.

Morantz, R. 1977. 19th century health reform and women: A program of self-help. In *Medicine Without Doctors,* ed. G. Risse, R. Numbers, and J. Leavitt. New York: Science History Publications.

Nagel, J. 1996. *American Indian ethnic renewal.* New York: Oxford University Press.

National Center for Health Statistics. 1993. Advance report of final mortality statistics, 1993. vol. 44, no. 7. Supplement 1996. Washington, D.C.: Department of Health and Human Services.

National Center for Policy Analysis. 1998. Creeping Clinton care. http://www.ncpa.org/health/pdh72.htm.

Nature program, "American Buffalo: Spirit of a Nation." http://www.pbs.org/wnet/nature/buffalo/nation.html.

Navarro, V. 1976. *Medicine under capitalism.* New York: Pro Dist.

Norgen, J. 1996. *The Cherokee cases: The confrontation of law and politics.* New York: McGraw-Hill, Inc.

Norman, Geoffrey 1995. The Cherokee: Two nations, one people. *National Geographic* 187 (5):72–97.

Oklahoma City Area Indian Health Service. 1995. Summary Sheets and Tables for the Cherokee Nation of Oklahoma.

Office of Technology Assessment. 1986. Indian health care. Washington, D.C.: GPO.

Public Health Service. 1986. Department of Health and Human Services. 42 CFR Part 36 Indian Health Services; Eligibility; Proposed Rule. Federal Register, vol. 51, no. 111: 21118–22. Tuesday, June 10, 1986.

Prucha, F. 1981. *Cherokee removal: The William Penn essays and other writings of Jeremiah Warts.* Knoxville: University of Tennessee Press.

Quirk, P. 1989. The cooperative resolution of policy conflict. *American Political Science Review* 83 (3):905–21.

Congressional Record. 1896. 54th Cong., 1st sess. 24 Feb. Vol. 28:2079.

Riessman, F., and D. Carroll. 1995. *Redefining self-help.* San Francisco: Jossey-Bass.

Riessman, F. and A. Gartner. 1984. *Self-help revolution.* New York: Human Sciences Press.

Robinson, D. and S. Henry. 1977. *Self-help and health: mutual aid for modern problems.* New York: Martin Robinson.

Royce, C. 1975. *The Cherokee Nation of Indians.* Chicago: Aldine Publishing Company.

Rubin, L. 1969. Maximum feasible participation: The origins, implications and present status. *The Annals of the American Academy of Political and Social Science* 385:14.

New York Times. 1997. Senate measure would deal blow to Indian rights. August 27. Pp. A1, A12.

Sidel, V. and R. Sidel. 1984. *Reforming medicine: lessons of the last quarter-century.* New York: Pantheon Books.

Snipp, C. 1989. *American Indians: The first of this land.* New York: Russell Sage Foundation.

Snyder, W. 1963. *Dependency in psychotherapy: A casebook.* New York: MacMillan.

Stanton, E. 1970. *Clients come last.* New York: Sage Publications.

Starr, E. 1921. *History of Cherokee Indians and their legends and folklore.* Oklahoma City: Warden Co.

Stewart, M. 1990. Expanding theoretical conceptualizations of self-help groups. *Social Science and Medicine,* vol. 21, no. 9.

Sullivan, T. 1984. *Resolving development disputes through negotiation.* New York: Plenum.

Susskind, L., and J. Cruishank. 1989. *Breaking the impasse: Consensual approaches to resolving public disputes.* New York: Basic Books.

Thomas, R. 1961. The Redbird Smith movement. In *Symposium on Cherokee and Iroquois culture,* ed. W. Fenton, and J. Gluck. Bureau of American Ethnology Bulletin 180, no. 16: 150–66. Washington, D.C.: Smithsonian Institution.

Tracey, P. 1996. Cherokee reconstruction in Indian Territory. *Journal of the West* 35 (3): 81–85.

Unrau, W. 1989. *Mixed-bloods and tribal dissolution.* Lawrence, Kans.: University Press of Kansas.

U.S. Bureau of the Census. 1993. *Table 9: Summary of general characteristics of American Indian, Eskimo, or Aleut persons and households.* General Population Characteristics: United States Summary. Washington, D.C.

U.S. Commission on Civil Rights. 1981. Indian tribes: A continuing quest for survival. Washington, D.C.: GPO.

U.S. Congress 1988a. United States. Congress. Senate. Select Committee on Indian Affairs. Senate bill S. 2382 Delaying the implementation of a certain rule affecting the provision of health services by the Indian Health Service: report to accompany S. 2382. 100th Congress. 2nd Session. Washington, D.C.: U.S. GPO.

U.S. Congress. 1988b. United States. Congress. Senate. Select Committee on Indian Affairs. Eligibility for health care services provided by Indian Health Service: Hearing before the Select Committee on Indian Affairs, United States Senate, 100th Congress, 2nd Session. Washington, D.C.: U.S. GPO.

U.S. Congress. 1992. United States. Congress. Senate. Select Committee on Indian Affairs. Indian health care improvement act of 1992: Report to accompany Senate Bill S. 2481, August 27, 1992. Washington, D.C.: U.S. GPO.

Wald, P. 1992. Terms of assimilation: Legislating subjectivity in the emerging nation. *Boundary 2* 19 (3): 77–104.

Waldman, C. 1985. *Atlas of the North American Indian.* New York: Facts on File Publications.

Washburn, C. 1869. *Reminiscences of the Indians.* Richmond.

Wilson, E. 1998. *Consilience: The unity of knowledge.* New York: Alfred A. Knopf.

Withorn, A. 1986. Helping ourselves. In *The sociology of health and illness: Its role in social care,* ed. D. Pancost, P. Parker, and C. Froland. New York: Sage Publications.

Witthof, J. 1961. Eastern woodlands community typology and acculturation. In *Symposium on Cherokee and Iroquois culture,* ed. W. Fenton, and J. Gluck. Bureau of American Ethnology Bulletin 180, no. 9. Washington, D.C.: Smithsonian Institution.

Wollstein, J. 1998. The Clinton health care disaster. http://www.seventhquest.com/isil.org/pamphlet/clinton.htm.

Woodward, G. S. 1963. *The Cherokees.* Norman: University of Oklahoma Press.

Young, M. 1996. Conflict resolution on the Indian frontier. *Journal of the Early Republic* 16 (spring): 1–19.

Zapka, J., and B. Estabrook. 1976. Medical self-care programs. *Health Care Management Review,* vol. 1: 75–81.

Index